Skinny **Bastard**

Skinny **Bastard**

A Kick-in-the-Ass

for Real Men Who Want to Stop Being Fat

and Start Getting Buff

by Rory Freedman and Kim Barnouin

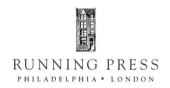

RUNNING PRESS

PHILADELPHIA • LONDON

9   8   7   6   5   4   3   2   1
Digit on the right indicates the number of this printing

Library of Congress Control Number: 2009922147

ISBN 978-0-7624-3934-8

Cover design by Bill Jones
Interior design by Maria Taffera Lewis
Edited by Jennifer Kasius
Typography: Dutch801, Helvetica Neue Light, and Boton

Running Press Book Publishers
2300 Chestnut Street
Philadelphia, Pennsylvania 19103-4371

Visit us on the web!
www.runningpress.com

Contents

For Bruce Friedrich—
you are truly one in a billion

Acknowledgments

As always, none of this would be possible without Tracy Silverman, Lauren Silverman, Talia Cohen, Laura Dail, Jennifer Kasius, Seta Zink, Craig Herman, Melissa Appleby, Peter Costanzo, Maria Taffera Lewis, Margarete Gockel, Victoria Gilder, Isabelle Bleecker, Bill Jones, David Steinberger, the entire sales team, and everyone else at Perseus and Running Press. Each and every one of you is a blessing.

Dina Aronson, MS, RD, you are as generous as you are brilliant— the words "thank you" seem awfully inadequate. Nonetheless, thank you, a thousand times over. And once more.

Special thanks to Dr. Neal Barnard and Dr. Hope Ferdowsian, for all you do and all you are.

Love and gratitude to Mikko Alanne, Lesley, Maya, and Tim Bailey, Chloé Jo Berman, James Costa, Sue Foley, Meri Freedman, Rick Freedman, Jackie Poper, Gretchen Ryan, Ari Solomon, Tim VanOrden, and Stephane and Jackson Barnouin.

Introduction

So you're fat. Big deal. Chances are, you haven't done so badly, despite the few extra lbs you're carting around. (Women are so amazing—we can be madly in love with a man, despite how he looks.) But don't kid yourself, pal: A hot-bodied man is a head-turner. So don't waste your money on a stupid sports car to get chicks; a woman who cares about what kind of car a man drives is a vapid, shallow whore. Invest in yourself. (A woman who cares about how a man looks is also a vapid, shallow whore. But at least you'll look good.) You have only one body to get you through this lifetime. So quit eating crap and abusing yourself! Even if you never look like Brad Pitt, if you're eating well and exercising, you'll be healthier, happier, and more confident. Chicks dig that shit.

So strap on a pair. It's time to get ripped.

(P. S. Just so we're all on the same page: We know men don't want to be skinny. We named the book *Skinny Bastard* because the title went well with our book for women, *Skinny Bitch*.)

Chapter 1

Give It Up

Okay. Use your head. You need to get healthy if you want to get buff. The first thing you need to do is give up your gross vices. Don't act surprised! You cannot keep eating the same shit and expect to lose weight. Or smoke. So don't even try some pathetic excuse like, "But if I quit smoking, I'll gain weight." No one wants to hear it. Cigarettes are for losers. They are so 1989 and totally uncool. Not only do they screw up your whole body chemistry, but they also kill your taste buds. It's no wonder you eat garbage. Smoking's out. Give it up. (If you chew tobacco, just put this book down now, because you probably don't even know how to read, anyway.)

Of course it is easier to socialize after you've had a few drinks. But being a fat pig will hinder you, sober or drunk. And habitual drinking equals fat-pig syndrome (not to mention pathetic-loser syndrome). Beer is for frat boys, not skinny bastards. It's high in sugar and makes you fat, bloated, and farty. Why do you think when kids go away to college they gain the "freshman fifteen"? Beer, duh. Alcohol isn't any better. It raises the level of hydrochloric acid in your stomach, wreaking havoc on the digestive process. If you suffer from poor digestion, then your food will not pass through your body properly. Hence, bloated fat-pig syndrome. To make matters worse, some alcohol (and nonorganic wines) still contains urethane, a cancer-causing chemical.[1] To boot, both beer and alcohol jack up your blood-sugar levels, which is bad for your bod. And don't kid yourself: When you have a hangover, you're bound to eat shit all day long.

We're not total killjoys—the occasional drink isn't gonna make or break anything. But even if it makes you feel like a priss, try trading your booze for organic red wine produced without sulfites. (Sulfites are additives used in food and wine to extend shelf life and fight bacteria growth. Asthma and allergic reactions can be triggered by sulfites. Even if wine is organic, that doesn't mean it is produced without sulfites. Read the label; it should say "no sulfites added" or "NSA." (Frey Vineyards makes organic, sulfite-free wines.) Organic red wine with NSA is rich in cancer-fighting antioxidants, can reduce risk of stroke, helps thin the blood, and has flavonoids, which lower cholesterol. Yes, organic red wine may be good for you. No, you should not drink a bottle by yourself every day. Alcohol can cause cancer, infectious diseases, cardiovascular disease, shrinking of the cerebral cortex, and can alter brain-cell function. And drunk men are gross. All kidding aside, don't be ashamed if you're an alcoholic; alcoholism is a disease. If you need help quitting drinking, call the Alcoholics Anonymous World Headquarters at (212) 870-3400 to find an AA meeting near you or visit www.alcoholics-anonymous.org.

Brace yourselves, boys: Soda is liquid Satan. It is the devil. It is garbage. There is nothing in soda that should be put into your body. For starters, soda's high levels of phosphorous can increase calcium loss from the body, as can sodium and caffeine.[2] You know what this means —bone loss, which may lead to osteoporosis (which does affect men). And the last time we checked, sugar, found in soda by the boatload, does not make you lose weight! Now don't go patting yourself on the back if you drink diet soda. That stuff is even worse. Aspartame (an ingredient commonly found in diet sodas and other sugar-free foods) has been blamed for a slew of scary maladies, like arthritis, fibromyalgia, Alzheimer's, lupus, multiple sclerosis, and diabetes.[3] When methyl alcohol, a component of aspartame, enters your body, it turns into formaldehyde. Formaldehyde is toxic and carcinogenic (cancer-causing).[4] Laboratory scientists use formaldehyde as a disinfectant or preservative. They don't fucking *drink* it. Perhaps you have a fat gut because you're preserving your fat cells with diet soda. The Food and Drug Administration has received more complaints about aspartame than any other ingredient to date.[5] Want more bad news? When aspartame is paired with carbs, it causes your brain to slow down its production of serotonin.[6] A healthy level of serotonin is needed to be happy and well-balanced. So drinking soda can make you fat, sick, and unhappy. Good luck with the ladies.

Unless you're from Mars, you've heard about the "eight glasses of water a day" thing. If you're filling up on 16 ounces of liquid Satan at a time, chances are you're not getting your 64 ounces of water a day. Water is vital for keeping your body clean and detoxified. It literally flushes out all the shit and toxins your body stores from your horrendous diet. You might be fat 'cause you don't crap enough. Drinking lots of water can help with the elimination process. Say goodbye to soda and hello to a sweet ass.

"Don't talk to me until I've had my morning coffee." Um . . . *pathetic*! Coffee is for pussies. Think about how widely accepted it has become that people *need* coffee to wake up. You should not *need* any-thing to wake up. If you can't wake up without it, it's because you are addicted to caffeine, sleep deprived, or a generally unhealthy slob. It may seem like the end of the world to give up your daily dose, especial-ly if you use Starbucks to go trolling for women. But it's not heroin, and you'll learn to live without it. Caffeine can cause headaches, diges-tive problems, irritation of the stomach and bladder, peptic ulcers, diarrhea, constipation, fatigue, anxiety, and depression. It affects every organ system, from the nervous system to the skin. Caffeine rais-es stress hormone levels, inhibits important enzyme systems that are responsible for cleaning the body, and sensitizes nerve reception sites.[7] It also raises blood pressure,[8] may cause an increased susceptibility to diabetes,[9] and may be linked to rheumatoid arthritis.[10] But don't go grabbing for the decaf. Coffee, whether regular or decaf, is highly acidic.[11] Acidic foods cause your body to produce fat cells to keep the acid away from your organs.[12] (Please, do not link this acid issue to cit-rus and other fruits. We discuss this in depth later; on pages 33-34.) So coffee equals fat cells. P. S. It also makes your breath smell like ass. Furthermore, coffee beans, like other crops, are grown with chemical pesticides. One insecticide, D-D-7, has been banned in the United

Give It Up

States but is still used by other countries from which we import coffee beans.[13] So every single morning, you are starting your day with a dose of poison. Add sugar or other artificial sweeteners, top it off with milk or cream, and you'll be fat forever. If you enjoy an occasional cup of coffee, fine. But if you need it, give it up.

A much better way to start the day is with a macho-looking cup of caffeine-free herbal tea—organic, of course. Decaffeinated green tea is like a wonder drug. Its anti-aging and antibacterial qualities are as renowned as its reputation for fighting cancer, combating allergies, and lowering blood pressure. But don't overdo it or you may be at an increased risk for kidney stones. Go to a coffeehouse, if you must. Just get a decaf organic herbal tea instead of coffee. Plus, if women see you drinking tea, they'll think you're smart and sensitive. Miss your caffeine jolt? Get a fresh-squeezed organic juice for an instant jumpstart. Once you are rid of your caffeine addiction, you will get totally high from fresh-squeezed juice.

Junk food will never go away. It becomes more alluring by the minute with laboratory-developed aromas, artificial flavors, chemical food colors, toxic preservatives, and heart-stopping hydrogenated oils. We know it's impossible to resist, but no one ever got buff on candy, chips, cookies, and ice cream. Use your head. Not only is junk food bogged down with saturated fats, sugars, hydrogenated oils, calories, and cholesterol, but it also contains enough chemical residues to take the hair off your balls. Ever heard of butylated hydroxyamisole (BHA) or butylated hydroxytoluene (BHT)? Most people haven't, even though these chemical preservatives are put in food or into the packaging.[14] The FDA doesn't require companies to divulge the presence of these beauties if they are used in packaging, though they can come into contact with the food you're eating. So your junk food has a shelf life of twenty-two years and will probably outlive your next two cars. Now before you decide you're so smart 'cause you only buy fat-free snacks, get a hold of yourself. Whenever you see the words "fat-free" or "low-fat," think of the words "chemical shit storm." Read the ingredients. Do you really think sugar or hydrogenated oils or eggs or milk won't make you fat? Puh-lease! By the way, sugar, like coffee, creates an acidic environment in your body.[15] You just learned that acidic foods cause your body to produce fat cells. So you do the math: sugar = fat. If you'd drag your ass to a health food store, you'd find aisle after aisle of "acceptable junk food"—guilt-free garbage that tastes so good, you'll do naked squats

Give It Up

in the parking lot. We are not saying you have to give up junk food to lose weight. You just have to trade your old junk food for new junk food. In Chapter 12, we provide an "acceptable junk food" list that'll give you a woody.

Are you a pill popper? Do you reach for over-the-counter medicine for every sniffle, sneeze, ache, and pain? Toughen up, pansy. Our bodies, when properly cared for, function as perfect machines. Our brains tell us when something is wrong by giving us pain or discomfort. When we pop pills to rid this "dis-ease," we are masking the symptoms without resolving the problem. Every time you take medicine, you interfere with your body's natural ability to heal itself. You are alleviating those intelligent responses that alert you to a problem and are sending false signals to your brain. If you have a headache, you might be tired, dehydrated, or suffering from a minor food allergy. Most likely, your body is having an adverse reaction to the unhealthy crap you're eating. Taking two aspirin is not the answer. If your nose is running, your body is trying to rid itself of something through your snot. But you, drama queen, take cold medicine to stop your runny nose. Now you've gone and fucked up everything. Medicine is made of chemicals. Never mind that the Food and Drug

Administration gives meds their stamp of approval. They also allow the use of aspartame. Use your own damn brain. Do you think putting chemicals in your body is good for you? Every medicine comes complete with a list of side effects. That means that taking medicine will make you feel better for the moment but will fuck up something else in your body. So suck it up. Stop interfering with Mother Nature.

(Obviously, if you are on prescribed medication, you need to consult a physician before discontinuing it.)

Give up the notion that you can be sedentary and still lose weight. Eating properly will dramatically improve your health, body, and all aspects of your life. But you've still gotta move your ass. Anyone with a brain can do the math: When done in conjunction with a good diet, exercise will make you lose weight faster than healthy eating alone. You don't need to spend seven days a week at the gym. In fact, you shouldn't, because too much exercise is bad for you (and men who work out too much look like fuckin' FREAKS). It can lead to dehydration, arthritis, osteoporosis, and injuries like strains, sprains, and fractures. Twenty minutes of cardiovascular a day, five days a week, is a good starting point. Then, after a couple of weeks, kick it up a notch. Depending on your fitness goals, you can increase your cardiovascular workout or add strength training to your routine, or both. Aim for working out in the morning, if you can. When we exercise, our elevated heart rates and deep breathing cause our "bodyminds" to enter a fat-burning mode that can last throughout the day.[16] Regardless of what time you work out, you'll soon become addicted to exercising. When we are active enough to break a sweat, our brains release endorphins[17] and feel-good opiates so that we grow to love this healthy activity. Exercise burns fat and calories, improves circulation, regulates crapping, defines muscles, builds strength, and detoxifies your body through sweating.[18] Plus, working out helps keep junk food cravings and savage appetites at bay. It's a win-win. Work out. (Oh, you probably don't care, but exercise also improves the sex drive and sexual function.)

Chapter 2

Carbs: The Truth

Never before has the United States seen such a ridiculous diet trend as the "low-carb" phenomenon. Every restaurant, grocery store, and fast-food chain caters to this utter nonsense. Even soda and beer companies have spent millions developing and marketing low-carb drinks. Everyone has jumped on the bandwagon, hoping to capitalize on the trend, whether it is healthy or not. Not.

Carbohydrates are compounds made up of carbon, hydrogen, and oxygen, and they are *vital* for providing energy for our bodies and brains. Without them, we would be comatose zombies. When we eat food, our bodies turn the carbohydrates into glucose for immediate energy and the rest is stored as glycogen for reserves.

Yet all carbs are not created equal. There are two types: simple (also referred to as refined) and complex. Simple carbohydrates suck and are as nutritionally beneficial as toilet paper. They are mostly made up of sugar, which releases too quickly, almost violently, into our bodies, causing "sugar highs" and then "crashes." This tends to leave us feeling hungry, so we eat more. On the other hand, complex carbohydrates are comprised of starch and fiber and release gradually, providing a steady source of energy. They make us feel full and satisfied and are easily broken down to release their energy. Shitty simple carbohydrates include white flour, white pasta (durum semolina), white rice, and white sugar. These are the bad boys that give all carbs a bad reputation. For some asinine reason, food manufacturers decided that we wouldn't buy their products unless they were white and soft. So they took natural grains, like brown rice and whole wheat, and stripped away all their nutrients, vitamins, and minerals to achieve the color and texture change. This refining process totally compromises the nutritional integrity of the food—all for appearances. So companies then add these nutrients back into their refined, milled foods and use terms like "enriched" or "fortified." But there's no use trying to fool with Mother Nature. Our bodies cannot absorb these added-in minerals with the same ease.[19] Tragically, most cereals, pastas, rice, bagels, breads, cookies, muffins, cakes, and pastries have been bastardized in this manner. Pay attention to how your body feels when you eat these foods. Chances are you'll notice moderate to severe mood swings and energy surges and losses.

Fear not. There are so many complex carbohydrates (Mother Nature is generous) that you'll never miss the simple shit. Bask in the glory of yams, sweet potatoes, barley, corn, brown rice, beans, hummus, lentils, quinoa (a grain, pronounced KEEN-wa), millet, and pasta made from brown rice, whole wheat, or vegetables. Bionaturae, Ancient Harvest, Eddie's Spaghetti, Lundberg Farms, Westbrae, Pastariso, and DeBoles Organic all carry these "good carb" pastas. Knock yourself out with breads and cookies and muffins made from whole wheat and other whole grains. (Whole grains are any that haven't been bleached, stripped, or refined and still possess all the nutrients from the original grain.) Food For Life has an amazing line of whole- and sprouted-grain breads, and Pacific Bakery and French Meadow Bakery carry organic breads that aren't too shabby, either. Don't forget the bounty of vegetables and fruits—complex carbs that supply the body with vitamins, minerals, and fiber.

Yeah, you heard us—fruit. Eat it. The most irritating thing about the low-carb craze is the resistance to eating fruit. We know it's not exactly

Carbs: The Truth

seen as "butch," but fruit is, quite possibly, the most perfect food in existence. It is unique in that it barely requires any work to be digested. High in enzymes, it effortlessly passes through the body, supplying carbohydrates, fiber, vitamins, minerals, fatty acids, amino acids, and cancer-fighting tannins and flavonoids. Because it is made up of mostly water, fruit hydrates the body and aids in cleansing, detoxifying, and eliminating (shitting). In other words, it's really fucking good for you.

So tell all your dumb-ass, misinformed friends: YOU CAN EAT BREAD AND FRUIT!

Chapter 3

Sugar Is for Candy-Asses

We know how difficult it is to stay away from sugar. But too bad. Man up, bitch.

Take a look around your kitchen and become aware of all the places sugar is lurking, waiting to strip you of your dignity. Probably in places you wouldn't ever expect to find it. Read the ingredients of your breakfast cereals, breads, crackers, junk foods, everything. Sugar is like crack, and food manufacturers know that if they add it to their products, you'll keep coming back for more.

What is it, exactly? In its simplest form, it is the juice from a sugar cane plant. A plant—that seems benign, right? And it is, in moderation, ingested in its raw, simplest form. But all the enzymes, fiber, vitamins, and minerals are destroyed during the refining process.[20] First, the cane is pressed to extract the juice. Then, the juice is boiled so that it will thicken and crystallize. Next, it is centrifuged, or spun,

Sugar Is for Candy-Asses

to remove the syrup. After that, the sugar is washed and filtered to remove any nonsugar materials and to decolorize it. (By the way, sugar filters are commonly made of charred animal bones. Nasty.) Finally, the sugar is dried and packaged. So you see, refined sugar has no nutritional value. And it's usually in foods that contain tons of fat, lots of useless calories, and loads of cholesterol. So, you become addicted to foods (because they contain sugar) that have a large amount of fat, saturated fat, hydrogenated oils, and calories. Refined sugar, a simple carbohydrate, has been linked to hypoglycemia, a weakened immune system, hyperactivity, attention deficit disorder, enlargement of the liver and kidneys, increase of uric acid in the blood, mental and emotional disorders, dental cavities, and an imbalance of neurotransmitters in the brain.[21] In addition, refined sugars make you *fat*. Excess amounts are stored in the liver as glycogen. But when the liver is too full, the excess amounts are returned to the bloodstream as fatty acids.[22] Guess where those end up? Your saggy, old-lady ass; your big, fat gut; and your man-boobs.

Not only is the sugar industry big business in America, but the United States is also the largest supplier of sugar-laden foods in the world. It's not enough to poison our own citizens. We have to fuck up the rest of the world, too, for a dime.

High fructose corn syrup is another badass that finds its way into tons of foods. Manufacturers love its versatility and put it in nearly everything: soda, beer, yogurt, energy bars, cookies, candies, breads, even frozen goods. High fructose corn syrup is processed more than sugar and is even sweeter. But it's a friend of the farmer because it's so cheap to produce. Like refined sugar, it has a negative, dramatic effect on our blood-sugar levels. According to studies conducted by the *American Journal of Clinical Nutrition*, diabetes and obesity are directly linked to eating refined sugar and high fructose corn syrup.[23]

We aren't telling you to give up dessert for the rest of your lives, so settle down crybaby. We're simply suggesting that you substitute natural, healthier alternatives for refined sugar. Blackstrap molasses, agave, and Stevia are better choices. Other good substitutes for refined sugar include evaporated cane juice, granulated cane juice, Sucanat, brown rice syrup, barley malt syrup, Rapadura sugar, Turbinado sugar, raw sugar, beet sugar, date sugar, maple syrup, maple syrup crystals, and molasses. (Some companies add lard to maple syrup or molasses to reduce foaming, so be sure you are buying 100 percent pure, organic products.) Don't shit yourself, but all of

Sugar Is for Candy-Asses

these natural sweeteners possess one or more of the following health benefits: enzymes, calcium, iron, potassium, protein, the B vitamins, magnesium, chromium, fiber, and folic acid. Some even contain complex carbohydrates.[24] We're not saying you should eat naturally sweetened cupcakes three meals a day. We're just saying that you *can* have your cake and eat it. Just use your head regarding the amount of sweets you consume. (Check out our "acceptable junk food list" starting on page 207 for some of our favorite goodies.)

Now that you've heard the good news about natural sweeteners, it's time to give up the all the bad ones. Obviously, refined sugar is bad for you, as is high fructose corn syrup. And in case you had your head up your ass during Chapter 1, STOP EATING AND DRINKING PRODUCTS THAT CONTAIN ASPARTAME! This includes diet sodas and sugar-free foods that have NutraSweet or Equal.

When aspartame was put before the FDA for approval, it was denied *eight* times. G.D. Searle, the company behind aspartame, tried to get FDA approval in 1973. Clearly, they weren't bothered by reports from neuroscientist Dr. John Olney and researcher Ann Reynolds (hired by Searle) that aspartame was dangerous.[25] Dr. Martha Freeman, a scientist from the FDA Division of Metabolic and

Endocrine Drug Products, declared, "The information submitted for review is inadequate to permit a scientific evaluation of clinical safety." Freeman recommended that until the safety of aspartame was proven, marketing the product should not be permitted.[26] Alas, her recommendations were ignored. Somehow, in 1974, Searle got approval to use aspartame in dry foods. However, it wasn't smooth sailing from there. In 1975, the FDA put together a task force to review Searle's testing methods. Task force team leader Phillip Brodsky said he "had never seen anything as bad as Searle's testing" and called test results "manipulated."[27] Before aspartame actually made it into dry foods, Olney and attorney and consumer advocate Jim Turner filed objections against the approval.[28]

In 1977, the FDA asked the U.S. attorney's office to start grand jury proceedings against Searle for "knowingly misrepresenting findings and concealing material facts and making false statements in aspartame safety tests." Shortly after, the U.S. attorney leading the investigation against Searle was offered a job by the law firm that was representing Searle. Later that same year, he resigned as U.S. attorney and withdrew from the case, delaying the grand jury's investigation. This caused the statute of limitations on the charges to run out, and the investigation was dropped. *And* he accepted the job with Searle's law firm.[29]

In 1980, a review by the Public Board of Inquiry set up by the FDA determined that aspartame should not be approved. The board said it had "not been presented with proof of reasonable certainty that aspartame is safe for use as a food additive." In 1981, new FDA Commissioner Arthur Hull Hayes was appointed. Despite the fact that three out of six scientists advised against approval, Hayes decided to overrule the scientific review panel and allow aspartame into limited dry goods. In 1983, he got it approved for beverages, even though the National Soft Drink Association urged the FDA to delay approval until further testing could be done. That same year, Hayes left the FDA amid charges of impropriety. The Internal Department of Health and Human Services was investigating Hayes for accepting gratuities from FDA-regulated companies. He went to work as a consultant for Searle's public relations firm. Interesting. The FDA finally urged Congress to prosecute Searle for giving the government false or incomplete test results on aspartame.[30] However, the two government attorneys assigned to the case decided not to prosecute. Later, they went to work for the law firm that represented Searle.

Fascinating. Despite recognizing ninety-two different toxic symptoms that result from ingesting aspartame, the FDA approved it for use, without restriction, in 1996.[31] Brilliant.

So many people have been sickened from this shit that there are aspartame victim support groups. Some of the ninety-two aspartame side effects listed by the FDA include abdominal pain, memory loss, nerve cell damage, migraines, reproductive disorders, mental confusion, brain lesions, blindness, joint pain, Alzheimer's, bloating, nervous system disorders, hair loss, food cravings, and weight gain.[32]

Aspartame is a $1 billion industry.[33] The National Justice League has filed a series of lawsuits against food companies using aspartame, claiming they are poisoning the public. In September 2004, a class-action lawsuit was filed for $350 million against NutraSweet and the American Diabetics Association. George W. Bush's Secretary of Defense Donald Rumsfeld is named in the suit for using political muscle to get aspartame approved by the FDA.[34] NutraSweet and Equal contain aspartame. When ingested, one of aspartame's ingredients, methyl alcohol, converts into formaldehyde, a deadly neurotoxin.[35] In addition to aspartame, Equal contains the amino acid phenylalanine. Phenylalanine occurs naturally in the brain. But high levels can increase the chance of seizures and lead to depression and schizophrenia.[36] There is no lesser of the two evils. NutraSweet and Equal are both bad. Sweet & Low is no saint, either. It is an artificial sweetener that contains saccharin, a coal-tar compound.[37] Stay away.

Because we're having so much fun, let's bash the shit out of Splenda, one of the newer sweeteners—especially since it had 60 percent of the consumer market for artificial sweeteners in 2006.[38] Splenda is made by chlorinating sugar, changing its molecular structure. The finished product is called sucralose. The makers of this poison tout its lack of calories and claim it's safe for diabetics. The FDA calls sucralose 98 percent pure. The other 2 percent contains small amounts of heavy metals, methanol, and arsenic.[39] Well, gee, at least it doesn't have calories. So what if it has a little arsenic? Sucralose has been found to cause diarrhea; organ, genetic, immune system, and reproductive damage; and swelling of the liver and kidneys.[40] What a splendid product! According to Dr. Joseph Mercola in the *Consumer Research* article "The Potential Dangers of Sucralose," "There is no clear-cut evidence that sugar substitutes are useful on weight reduction. On the contrary, there is some evidence that these substances may stimulate appetite."[41]

Not only have multiple class-action lawsuits been filed, but the president of the National Sugar Association and the manufacturer of Equal also had their panties in a bunch over Splenda. They each filed suit, claiming that Splenda manufacturers are misleading consumers into thinking the product is natural when it is "a highly processed chemical compound."[42] (Don't think that the giants behind artificial sweeteners and the sugar industry suddenly started caring about public health. Splenda is just totally screwing up their sales. But even executive director for the Center for Science in the Public Interest, Dr. Michael F. Jacobson, who normally criticizes the National Sugar Association, had to agree: "Advertising and labeling, whether for products that are healthful or unhealthful, should be truthful and not misleading.")[43] The makers of Splenda settled both lawsuits. With the Equal lawsuit, it was reported that settlement talks began after jurors requested a calculator and white board, indicating they were going to rule against Splenda and were trying to figure out a dollar amount.[44]

Clearly, artificial sweeteners and refined sugars are bad for many reasons. Here's one more. We have a delicate balancing act occurring in our bodies at all times—pH balance. Basically, everything we eat has its own pH balance. When food is digested, it leaves an acid or alkaline "ash" in the body, depending on the food's mineral content. Surprise, surprise: Artificial sweeteners are highly acid forming. (Coffee, excessive protein, meat, pasteurized dairy, refined sugars, and fatty foods are, too.)[45]

When our bodies get too acidic, we are much more prone to illness.[46] Sometimes, we don't even know we're sick until it's too late. But we can notice mild maladies, like skin problems, allergies, headaches, or colds.[47] Or, we can experience major trauma—severe damage to our thyroid glands, liver, and adrenal glands.[48] If our pH balance becomes too acidic, our bodies will react to protect themselves. To neutralize the acid, they will take alkalizing minerals from our reserves. If our reserves are low, the body will withdraw minerals from our bones and muscles.[49] If that doesn't scare you, consider this: Cancer cells thrive in acidic environments.[50] Cancer loves sugar.

Now, logically, it would seem that citrus fruits are acidic, but actually, when they enter the body, they are alkalizing. We know this appears to defy common sense because they seem like they'd be acidic. But they contain potassium and calcium, which are alkalizing minerals. They also have a high percentage of alkaline salts. Nearly all fruits, vegetables, and legumes are alkaline when they enter the body.[51] Other alkalizing foods are sea vegetables, miso, soybeans, and tofu.

Fruit, good. Natural sweeteners, good. Refined sugars, bad. Artificial sweeteners, bad. Any questions?

Chapter 4

Meat: Rotting, Decaying, Decomposing Flesh

The High-Protein/Low-Carb Pile of Bullshit

The Atkins diet. Hmm. Eat the flesh of dead cows, dead pigs, and dead chickens. Avoid fresh fruit. You are a total moron if you think the Atkins diet will get you ripped. Or, you are a gluttonous pig who wants to believe you can eat cheeseburgers all day long and lose weight. Perhaps you weren't listening the first time: You need to get healthy if you want to get buff! Eating carcasses all day while avoiding fresh fruit and whole grains is a recipe for disaster. Of course, if you stop eating refined carbohydrates, you will lose weight. That's the part of the Atkins Diet that actually works. However, most of the weight you lose is water weight. You see, when our bodies metabolize protein (found in high amounts in meat and dairy), nitrogen waste is released in the form of urea. Urea is toxic and must be passed out of the body through urine. So the high-protein diet isn't ridding your body of fat. It's just serving as a diuretic—making you pee more to flush out the toxic urea.[52] But whether you lose this piss weight initially is inconsequential. You will be a fat, unhealthy, smelly slob if you live this way.

Trendy diets like Atkins become popular for one reason: They hide behind scientific jargon that *seems* to make sense and allow you to eat unhealthy, fattening foods as long as you avoid carbs. You believe in these diets because you want to. But eating a typical high-protein diet can increase your daily fat intake by about 8–18 grams, more than double your cholesterol intake, and reduce your fiber intake by approximately 500 percent![53] Losing weight is supposed to make you healthier, not rob you of your vitality. Eating a high-protein diet is an inefficient, ineffective way to lose weight, and it increases risk for cancer, high blood pressure, gout, osteoporosis, muscular fatigue, depression, and some seriously badass breath.[54] Most Americans eat twice as much protein as necessary,[55] which has sent obesity, heart disease, and cancer rates soaring over the past fifty years. When you eat large amounts of animal protein and saturated fats and do not eat whole grains, vegetables, and fresh fruits, there is no fiber to bind all of the toxins and fat together to be eliminated from your body. You will eventually do an incredible amount of harm to yourself. And you're in jeopardy of developing kidney stones,[56] one of the most painful conditions known to man. If you're already at risk for reduced kidney function (tens of millions of Americans are and don't even know it), you may be causing serious mayhem.[57] By the time your blood shows the effects, it will be too late to reverse the damage. Diabetics are in even worse trouble with a high-protein diet because they are already at a higher risk of kidney disease to begin with. In a study involving 1,500 patients with diabetes, most had lost more than half of their kidney function because of a high intake of animal protein.[58] A study commissioned by Dr. Atkins himself found his dieters suffering from constipation, halitosis, headaches, and hair loss![59]

Who Wants to Live? Anybody? Bueller?

Don't care about your kidneys? What about your other organs? A study of more than 500,000 individuals linked the consumption of meat to pancreatic cancer.[60] While pancreatic cancer is relatively uncommon, the survival statistics are very grim.[61] Another study of nearly 50,000 men linked meat-eating to colon cancer.[62] People who eat red meat just once a week have a 38 percent greater risk; those who eat poultry just once a week have a 55 percent greater risk![63] Another recent study found meat-eaters at 67 percent higher risk for colorectal cancer, despite any genetic factors.[64] In terms of mortality, colorectal cancer is the United States' second most common cancer (and the fourth most common, worldwide).[65] Unsurprisingly, studies showed the intake of fruits, vegetables, whole grains, and legumes to be preventative and protective for multiple cancers.[66]

Don't care about cancer and just want to lose weight? (Dumbass.) The American Cancer Society conducted a study over a ten-year period with nearly 80,000 people trying to lose weight. Participants who ate meat three times a week or more gained substantially more weight than participants who avoided meat and consumed more vegetables.[67] Also, studies published in *The Journal of Clinical Nutrition* and *The New England Journal of Medicine* stated that meat eaters are much more likely to be overweight than vegetarians.[68]

P. S. Studies show that those who consume diets high in saturated fat and cholesterol but low in fruits, veggies, and fiber are at higher risk for Alzheimer's.[69]

Common Sense, Bitches

Before you start spouting off information you've been brainwashed with about evolution and the food chain, read on. Yes, humans have a high level of intelligence. Yes, we created weapons for hunting and fire for cooking. Yes, we found a way to mass-produce animals for consumption. However, if you study animals in the wild, you will note that they do not rely on anything other than their natural hunting ability, speed, strength, claws, teeth, and jaws. They have no tools or weapons. Now look at yourself. Look at your flimsy fingernails in comparison to an eagle's talons. Look at your flat, blunt, closely spaced teeth compared to a lion's sharp, knife-like, gap-spaced teeth. (The gaps ensure that meat doesn't get stuck between the animals' teeth.)[70] Compare your speed and agility to that of a tiger. Compare the strength of your jaw to a wolf's. Imagine yourself trying to run after an animal, catch it, and kill it using your bare hands, finger-nails, teeth, and jaws. Don't kid yourself: You'd get your ass kicked. And even if you were successful, envision yourself eating the kill without the aid of an oven and silverware.[71] Yes, the human brain allows us to stay removed from the process of hunting. But does this mean we are "evolved" and "intelligent" and should be eating animal flesh just because we can? Man's brain and "intelligence" also created alcohol, cigarettes, and drugs. Should we drink, smoke, and use just because we can?

Many meat eaters credit eating meat for our evolution from cavemen into what we are now. Scientific evidence suggests it's simply not true; many anthropologists believe we descended from vegetarian ancestors.[72] But even if eating meat did help us to evolve, look at what we evolved *from*. We looked like friggin' apes and had massive heads, strong jaws, and brute strength. Man was a different animal then.

The second we put food in our mouths, the digestion process begins, thanks to our saliva. Guess what? Our alkaline saliva is not meant to break down animal flesh; carnivores have acid saliva, perfectly designed for the task.[73] And hydrochloric acid, essential for

Meat: Rotting, Decaying, Decomposing Flesh

digesting carcass, is secreted in very small amounts in our stomachs. However, the stomachs of carnivores have ten times more hydrochloric acid than ours.[74] Our enzymes, digestive tracts, and organs are all different from those found in carnivores. Like it or not, our kidneys, colon, and liver are ill-equipped to process animal flesh. Compared with carnivores, our intestines are very long, so food that doesn't get adequately processed becomes clogged in our intestines. Animals quickly pass food through their digestive systems, but we have food rotting, decomposing, and fermenting in our intestinal tracts and colons; hence the need for colonics.[75] You don't see many tigers getting colonics, do you? You do see them napping, though. Even though their bodies are designed to digest meat, animals generally sleep all day while doing so because it is such a taxing process. Genetically and structurally, we are designed to thrive on plant foods.[76] William C. Roberts, M.D., editor of the *American Journal of Cardiology*, said, "When we kill animals to eat them, they end up killing us because their flesh, which contains cholesterol and saturated fat, was never intended for human beings, who are natural herbivores."[77] Natural carnivores living in the wild do not suffer from heart disease, cancer, or diabetes—our biggest killers. And whether it is "lean meat" or a "skinless chicken breast," animal fat is still animal fat. Don't be fooled by terms coined by the meat industry. Your body can't handle animal fat, so it settles like lumpy shit all over your body and sends you to an early grave.

Old MacDonald
Had a Very Different Farm

Of the ten billion land animals slaughtered each year in America for human consumption, nearly all of them come from factory farms. Factory farms that raise cattle, pigs, chickens, egg-laying hens, veal calves, or dairy cows have an enormous amount of animals in a very small space. There are no vast meadows or lush, green pastures. In the cases of chickens and egg-laying hens, the animals are confined inside buildings, where they are packed in on top of each other. Egg-laying hens are crammed into cages so small they are unable to spread their wings, and their feet and flesh get mangled against the wire mesh. This overcrowded, stressful environment causes chickens to peck at each other, so their beaks are chopped off their faces using a hot knife. Pigs and cows are imprisoned in stalls so small they are unable to turn around or lie down comfortably. Cattle are subject to third-degree branding burns and having their testicles and horns ripped out. Pigs also suffer from castration, in addition to the mutilation of their ears, tails, and teeth. They all live in the filth of their own urine, feces, and vomit with infected, festering sores and wounds. To keep animals alive in these unsanitary conditions, farmers must give them regular doses of antibiotics. Of the 50 million pounds of antibiotics made in the United States each year,[78] *70 percent* are administered to farm animals,[79] causing antibiotic resistance in the humans who eat them.

This Shit Is Crazy

Eating meat has been linked to obesity; cancer; liver, kidney, lung, and reproductive disorders; birth defects; miscarriages; and nervous system disorders.[80] For shits and giggles, we've compiled a partial list of what's in meat, poultry, seafood, and dairy: benzene hexachloride (BHC), chlordane, dichlorodiphenyltrichloroethane (DDT), dieldrin, dioxin, heptachlor, hexachlorobenzene (HCB), and lindane.[81] American farmers started using chemical pesticides in the late 1800s and were initially thrilled with the results. However, it was eventually noticed that pesticides were killing those who were most exposed to them: farmers, field workers, and animals. In 1972, the Environmental Protection Agency banned DDT.[82] But the pesticides that followed were even worse. BHC is 19 times more carcinogenic than DDT, chlordane 4 times more, dieldrin 47 to 85 times more, HCB 23 times more, and heptachlor 15 to 30 times more.[83] By the late 1980s, of the 450 endangered animal species, more than half were threatened with extinction.[84] The government finally called for a ban on the production and use of other pesticides. But this didn't stop these pesticides from reaching our food supply. Companies were allowed to use up their enormous stockpiles of these pesticides by selling them to countries outside of America. (Apparently, it was acceptable to poison people and animals, as long as they weren't American.) These countries used the pesticides on their crops, which were then imported into the United States.[85] Brilliant, huh? And, banned or not, once they have entered the soil or water, pesticides can still poison for decades.[86] One widely used pesticide, glufosinate, whose residues have been found in U.S.

waters and food supplies, causes hormonal and brain damage.[87] A University of Iowa study found that nearly 56 percent of children living on hog farms had asthma.[88] Pregnant women living in agricultural regions in California are more likely to have babies with severe birth defects.[89] Farmers who use large amounts of insecticides, pesticides, and herbicides (and their families) seem to have it worse than everyone:

* In Nebraska, farmers had a higher mortality rate from leukemia than any other working group.[90]

* Cotton farmers from Minnesota to Texas have steadily increasing leukemia rates.[91]

* Farmers in Wisconsin and Iowa have increased risk of non-Hodgkin's lymphoma.[92]

* Washington farmers have a higher incidence of soft-tissue sarcomas.[93]

* Washington ranchers and Minnesota farmers have higher mortality rates from central nervous system diseases and brain cancer.[94]

   Sadly, the list goes on and on.

   In his book, *Diet for a Poisoned Planet*, David Steinman reports that of all the toxic chemicals found in food, 95 to 99 percent come from meat, fish, dairy, and eggs.[95] He also reveals that many of the governmental safety tests performed don't even detect many chemicals and pesticides. The Food and Drug Administration's own Total Diet Study found that bacon had 124 different residues from pesticides, chemicals, and other industrial pollutants; bologna and other luncheon meats had 136; fast-food hamburgers had 285 residues; fast-food chicken nuggets had 184; hot dogs had 207; and ground beef had 180.[96] In butter, the residue of more than 384 pesticides and industrial pollutants was detected, 171 in cheddar cheese, 173 in cream cheese, 168 in processed American cheese, and 160 in Swiss cheese.[97] Sick, sick, sick! In comparison, meat contains 14 times more pesticides than plant foods; dairy has 5 times more pesticides than plant foods. Based on his review of USDA meat inspection reports, Steinman also estimates that "50 percent of animal foods could easily be contaminated with carcinogenic pesticides."[98] The United States alone uses *1.5 billion pounds* of pesticides every year![99] That, our pathetic contamination sampling process, and our use of growth hormones has caused the European Economic Community to reject our meat exportations on numerous occasions.[100]

Meat: Rotting, Decaying, Decomposing Flesh

Many animals are even given drugs laced with the most toxic form of arsenic.[101] Arsenic! Chemical pesticides are often sprayed directly onto the skin of animals to ward off parasites, insects, rodents, and fungi. In addition, these animals are given food treated with pesticides. On factory farms, bigger is better. More meat, milk, and eggs mean more money for the farmers. So to grow them larger or produce more, animals are given steroids and growth hormones. But what is happening to the people who eat these fattened animals? Young girls are experiencing early onset of puberty at epidemic proportions. Many scientists attribute this to all of the hormones in chicken, meat, and milk that are forced upon children. Basically, every time you consume factory-farmed chicken, beef, veal, pork, eggs, or dairy, you are eating antibiotics, pesticides, steroids, and hormones. This is worth repeating: *Every time you consume factory-farmed chicken, beef, veal, pork, eggs, or dairy, you are eating antibiotics, pesticides, steroids, and hormones.*

Now you might be thinking, "Who cares about all this pesticide-cancer shit? I just want to get buff!" Ever heard women complaining about gaining weight from going on The Pill or from having fertility treatments? Well, eating animals that are given hormones has the same effect as if you were taking these directly. According to Dr. Paula Baillie-Hamilton, author of *The Body Restoration Plan*, antibiotics alone can account for weight gain in animals.[102] She also states that the toxic chemicals used in food production are fattening. Whether it's the pesticides used for growing crops or the chemicals given to animals to fatten them up, they alter the body's metabolism in a way that causes weight gain. Having studied animals and humans, she discovered that low doses of toxic chemicals increased appetite, slowed metabolism, decreased ability to burn stored fat, and reduced ability to exercise.[103] The FDA lists approximately 1,700 drugs approved for use in animal feed. Of these approved drugs, approximately 300 include "weight gain" in their description.[104] However, in *Animal Factories*, Jim Mason and Peter Singer disclose an estimate of 20,000 to 30,000 different drugs actually being used.[105]

We constantly hear gym-rats bragging, "I don't eat any red meat. I just eat chicken." Well now you know: Chicken is just as bad for you as cow or pig. In fact, it might even be worse. According to a survey by the National Research Council, one chicken manufacturing plant had 90 percent of its poultry contami-

Meat: Rotting, Decaying, Decomposing Flesh

nated with salmonellosis.[106] Ninety fucking percent! Nasty. And according to the *American Journal of Epidemiology*, eating chicken (and fish) is linked to colon cancer. Researchers examined the eating habits of 32,000 men and women over a six-year period and then monitored emerging cancer cases for the next six years. "Among participants who generally avoided red meat but who ate white meat less than once per week, colon cancer risk was 55 percent higher than for those who avoided both kinds of meat. Those who had white meat at least once per week had more than three-fold higher colon cancer risk."[107]   Researchers at the National Cancer Institute found grilled chicken to have high levels of heterocyclic amines (HCA), carcinogens that are formed when animal proteins are heated. With 480 nanograms of heterocyclic amines per gram, grilled chicken registered 15 times higher than beef.[108] But don't go trading your chicken for beef. HCAs can form from cooking chicken, beef, pork, and fish, and whether you're grilling, frying, or broiling. Grilling or broiling over a flame also produces polycyclic aromatic hydrocarbons (PAH), more carcinogens.[109] So don't think cooking dead animals over an open flame makes you the grill-master; it makes you the cancer-master.

And don't be lulled into a false sense of security that our government keeps food safe. News of the avian influenza epidemic came and went, but this disease is very real and can run rampant in poultry flocks.

Unfortunately, our waters aren't any better than our land. Yes, some fish contain essential fatty acids and vitamins, minerals, and protein. But you can easily get all these nutrients from flaxseeds; pumpkin, sesame, and sunflower seeds; nuts; soybeans; fruits; vegetables (especially leafy greens); soy products; and whole grains. Fish and other seafood contain high levels of contaminants from industrial and environmental pollutants, waste products, and pesticide residues from farms. Also present in fish and seafood are high levels of mercury and PCBs, which are well absorbed by the body. Other notables are BHC, chlordane, DDT, dieldrin, heptachlor, and dioxin.[110] These chemicals can cause neurotoxicity, which impairs a person's mental state and ability. The human body contains acetylcholine, a naturally occurring chemical that helps impulses pass from nerve to nerve. Once the impulse is passed, the chemical is no longer needed and is actually harmful if it remains. So our bodies produce an enzyme, cholinesterase, which rids us of the unwanted acetylcholine. Pesticides inhibit our ability to pro-duce cholinesterase, which causes a buildup of the now-dangerous acetylcholine.[111] Mercury, a suspected carcinogen, can alter immune function, raise blood pressure, cause blindness or paraly-sis, increase the chance of cardiac mortality, and is known to reduce virility.[112] It can also inflict permanent brain damage on fetuses, infants, and children.

Appetizing, huh? Have some mercury poisoning with your ahi tuna. How about some trichinosis with your pork? Don't forget a side of salmonella with your eggs or chicken! We certainly don't want to leave out an order of mad cow disease! Think about what you've been eating. What we call salmon, hamburger, steak, chick-en, bacon, sausage, ham, roast beef, salami, bologna, turkey, hot dog, and duck are actually decomposing, rotting animal carcass. Bon appétit!

Man Up

Closing your eyes to the problem will not make it go away. You don't want to *see* it, but you'll *eat* it? So, yeah, if you want to be a

Skinny **Bastard**

Skinny Bastard, you've got to be a vegetarian—someone who doesn't eat dead animals or seafood. Quit whining. We weren't raised by hippie-crunchy-granola parents on vegetarian communes. Growing up, we both ate meat all day, every day. We scoffed at tofu and spit on vegetables. Really. Kim's addictions included such delicacies as corned beef hash, canned Vienna sausages, and daily Big Macs. Every single day in 1992, Rory ate a ham, egg, and cheese sandwich for breakfast, followed by a bacon double cheeseburger, fries, and a soda for lunch. Dinner was always a dead chicken, fish, cow, or pig. So before you say, "I could never give up meat," realize that nearly every single vegetarian on the planet said those same words. So shut it, pussy. And know that there are a ton of strong, manly, ass-kicking warriors who are vegetarians *and* professional athletes. (We list a few on pages 106–108, but don't skip ahead—wait for it.)

Now, some of you may be ready to explode. Certainly, when you bought this book, the last thing you expected was to be told that you should stop eating animals. But just because you didn't expect it or because it goes against what you've believed your whole life, it doesn't make the information any less accurate or

Meat: Rotting, Decaying, Decomposing Flesh

valuable. Simmer down. Step back for a second. Ask yourself why you're angry. Wait sixty seconds. Now ask yourself again—usually the first time you're not able to see the truth. Chances are you're angry because we've revealed a huge pile of shit that you didn't want to see. You were perfectly happy eating burgers and chicken and bacon, and the last thing you wanted was to know exactly what you were eating all these years. You were perfectly happy thinking these foods were healthy, or at least "okay in moderation." Now that you know all this, you won't be able to look at food the same way. Now that you know all this, you might actually have to change! And some of you would rather numb out, hate us, or hold on to your old, unhealthy ways than change. Well, we hope you'll take on the challenge of change. Because we both know from experience that abstaining from animal products is the best thing you can do for yourself. But don't take it from us, take it from the American Dietetic Association, the world's largest organization of nutrition professionals. After extensively reviewing all the scientific studies on vegetarian diets, they found that vegetarians have lower rates of obesity, diabetes, heart disease, high blood pressure, and cancer (all the top killers) than meat-eaters.[113] In other words, just so we're clear: vegetarians are healthier than meat eaters.

If you absolutely cannot, will not, dare not believe what we're saying about meat, or you simply don't want to stop eating these foods—fine. Just don't throw the baby out with the bathwater! You know there's other useful information in this book. So don't use this as an excuse to dismiss everything else you've learned since you started reading it. Just ignore the stuff you simply can't abide by and incorporate what you can. No need to be a drama queen about the whole thing.

Chapter 5

The Dairy Disaster

Go suck your mother's tits. Go on. Suck your mother's tits. You think this is ridiculous? It is. Get ready to use your head.

When a woman gives birth, her body produces milk, and she nurses her child. Breast milk can grow an 8-pound newborn into a 24-pound toddler. Sounds pretty fattening, huh? It is. By design, it is intended to allow for the biggest growth spurt of a person's entire life. Breast milk alone can accommodate for a 300 percent weight gain in a twelve-month period. When her child is anywhere from 12 to 24 months old, a mother stops breastfeeding. Her milk dries up. The child will never drink breast milk ever again.

Cows, like all mammals, are much the same. Their bodies produce milk only when they give birth. Contrary to popular belief, they do not need to be milked—ever. Their udders, like women's breasts,

exist even when there is no milk in them. There is one major difference, however. Cows' milk, by design, grows a 90-pound calf into a
2,000-pound cow over the course of two years.[114] It allows calves to
double their birth weight in forty-seven days and leaves their four
stomach chambers feeling full. Sounds even more fattening than
human milk, right? It is. It should be. Cows are bigger than humans.
And the inner workings of their bodies are completely different from
ours, which they should be. They are cows. We are humans. Duh.

Humans need the enzyme lactase to digest lactose (the sugar
found in dairy). However, between the ages of 18 months and 4
years, we lose 90 to 95 percent of this enzyme. The undigested lactose and the acidic nature of pasteurized milk encourage the growth
of bacteria in our intestines.[115] All this contributes to a greater risk of
cancer because cancer cells thrive in acidic conditions.[116] Got mucus?
Dairy products produce mucus and often, the body will develop a
cold or "allergies" to fight the dairy invasion.[117]

Mother Nature is no fool. All species, including ours, have just
what we need to get by. She did not intend for grownups to suck their
mothers' tits. We don't need our mothers' milk as adults, just like
grown cows don't need their mothers' milk anymore. We are the only

species on the planet that drinks milk as adults. We are also the only species on the planet that drinks the milk of another species. We could be putting gorilla milk on our cereal or having zebra milk and cookies. Why cows' milk? Using the animal that produces the largest quantity of milk but is more easily housed than an elephant means more money for farmers. It has nothing to do with health or nutrition. Again, it all comes back to money. The dairy industry is a multibillion-dollar industry based on brilliant marketing and the addictive taste of milk, butter, and cheese. It has convinced most doctors, dieticians, consumers, and government agencies that we *need* cows' milk.

Bone Loss, Cancer, and Illness, Oh My!

We have been told our whole lives, "You need milk to grow. Without milk, your bones will break. If you don't drink milk, you'll get osteoporosis. You need the calcium." *Bullshit*.

The Harvard Nurses' Health Study followed more than 72,000 women over the course of twelve years. And guess what? Milk was **not shown** to have a protective effect on bones![118] Researchers at Yale did a study using thirty-four surveys from sixteen countries found in twenty-nine research publications. They reported the same findings.[119] Americans are among the top consumers of dairy products in the world. So if dairy does what the dairy industry claims, we should have among the lowest rates of osteoporosis in the world, right? According to *The Journal of Gerontology*, American women over fifty have among the highest rates of hip fractures in the world. The only countries with higher rates are those that consume more milk![120] (Sorry for the girl-talk here. Because men have larger, stronger bones than women, you have a better likelihood of avoiding osteoporosis.[121] So while it does exist in men, it's just more prevalent in women, hence the better-developed studies. But don't go celebrating: 2 million men have it, 12 million are at risk, and countless more cases are unreported or undiagnosed.)[122] There is a very clear and strong association between bone fracture rates and the consumption of animal protein.[123] If you're not outraged, you aren't paying attention. The whole reason we douse ourselves with dairy is because it "strengthens bones." But scientific studies show that it does the exact opposite! If you aren't seething mad right now, check your pulse. You've been living a lie your whole life so that a few people could make money! (P. S. Consuming high amounts of dairy blocks iron

The Dairy Disaster

absorption, contributing to iron deficiency.)[124]

Cows' milk has one of the lowest absorption rates of all calcium sources.[125] One reason is its high protein content. A study showed vegans (people who abstain from animal products, including dairy) and omnivores having the same blood levels of calcium, even though the omnivores ingested *twice as much calcium*.[126] Yes, milk is high in calcium, but it's not an efficient source for it. Remember in Chapter Three when we talked about how sugar creates an acidic environment in the body? Well, so do dairy products. And this acidity causes an excretion of calcium in the urine.[127] Loss of calcium . . . osteoporosis.

According to *The China Study*'s Dr. T. Colin Campbell, dairy can be blamed for all sorts of madness. Dr. Campbell attended Cornell on a PhD scholarship, authored more than three hundred research papers, and has *four decades* of high-level research experience. So *The China Study* is, um, a little more intellectual than our book. It's basically the most comprehensive study of diet and nutrition ever conducted in history—spanning over twenty years time; citing from more than 750 references; and partnering Cornell University, Oxford University, and the Chinese Academy of Preventative Medicine. So what does this Holy Grail of nutrition say about dairy? That it can cause heart disease; diabetes; obesity; osteoporosis; kidney stones; cataracts; macular degeneration; multiple sclerosis; Alzheimer's; and prostate, colon, and rectal cancer![128] Dairy products have been linked to a host of other problems, too, including acne, anemia, anxiety, arthritis, attention deficit disorder, attention deficit hyperactivity disorder, fibromyalgia, headaches, heartburn, indigestion, irritable bowel syndrome, joint pain, poor immune function,[129] and ovarian cancer.[130] (Tell the ladies in your life.) Please, read this list again. Slowly. Let each one sink in. Are you pissed now?

Understandably, life is busy and you may not take the time to read *The China Study* right now. Well at some point soon, you really, really should. It's absolutely the most compelling, well-researched, in-depth book on nutrition we've ever come across. In the meantime, we're gonna give you just one of the many pertinent Cliff's Notes of *The China Study*: Dr. Campbell started a laboratory program to investigate protein's role in the development of cancer. Eventually, due to his diligent, precise, and careful practices, his research received funding for an extraordinary twenty-seven years from the National Institute of Health, the American Cancer Society, and the American Institute for Cancer Research (among others). In this time, he discov-

The Dairy Disaster

ered that protein did indeed have an effect on cancer. "What protein consistently and strongly promoted cancer? Casein, which makes up 87 percent of cow's milk protein, promoted all stages of the cancer process."[131]

There are three stages of cancer he's referring to: initiation, promotion, and progression. Dr. Campbell likens the stages to planting a lawn. "Initiation is when you put the seeds in the soil, promotion is when the grass starts to grow, and progression is when the grass gets completely out of control, invading the driveway, the shrubbery, and the sidewalk." Chemical carcinogens (byproducts of industrial processes) are usually what *initiate* normal cells to transform or mutate into cancer-prone cells. *Promotion* is when the cells "multiply until they become a visibly detectable cancer." And *progression* occurs when the cancer cells grow and spread.[132] Let us repeat: Casein, a milk protein, *promoted all three stages of cancer growth*. Incredibly interesting: His studies showed that exposure to toxic chemicals initiated cancer growth. But the cancer remained dormant and wasn't of issue. However, with the introduction of casein (milk protein), all that changed.[133]

According to two major Harvard studies, men who drink milk have a 30–60 percent greater cancer risk then those who avoid dairy.[134] And not just any cancer, but cancer of the co-co-co-cock. Prostate cancer is the most commonly diagnosed cancer in American men.[135] And one of the most consistent, specific links between diet and prostate cancer is dairy.[136] Honestly, if you aren't seeing red *now*, you're a lost cause.

Please go back and reread Dr. Campbell's credentials and the background information about *The China Study* once more. Acknowledge that *The China Study* isn't some hole-filled, half-baked, fluff piece, but that it's the real deal. Now get on board. Seriously. This is no joke. This is literally a matter of life and death. Do not dismiss this information just because it seems outlandish and hard to believe. Or just because your doctors and schoolteachers told you otherwise. According to a Senate investigation, doctors receive *less than three hours* of nutritional training in medical school![137] And unsuspecting teachers are puppets whose strings are pulled by the dairy industry. The dairy industry is a for-profit, commercial business, just like Pepsi or McDonald's. Imagine, however, if Pepsi or McDonald's were allowed to provide schools with educational mate-rials regarding nutrition. Unimaginable, right? Because more than likely, soda and Big Macs would be touted as important dietary sta-

The Dairy Disaster

ples. It'd probably sound a little something like this: "Pepsi has water in it, and it's vital to drink eight glasses of water a day. Big Macs are high in protein, and protein is an important component of any diet." We'd never stand for that, right? But we stand for the dairy industry—a for-profit enterprise—providing lesson plans, educational kits, posters, videos, and teaching guides to thousands of schools![138] And we allow them to sell milk at practically every school in the country! Doctors and teachers aren't dimwits or villains. They're just like the rest of us. It has been so ingrained into each one of us that "milk does a body good," that no one would ever think to question it. (Last chance to prove you're alive and well . . . swear your ass off, please!)

And because we've *all* been brainwashed, our children suffer. According to the Physicians Committee for Responsible Medicine (PCRM), "Insulin-dependent diabetes (Type 1 or childhood-onset) is linked to consumption of dairy products. Epidemiological studies of various countries show a strong correlation between the use of dairy products and the incidence of insulin-dependent diabetes. Researchers in 1992 found that a specific dairy protein sparks an autoimmune reaction, which is believed to be what destroys the insulin-producing cells of the pancreas."[139]

A Tall Glass of
Bovine Growth Hormone

Let's pretend for a moment that cows' milk is healthy for humans. Even if it were—it's not—but even if it were, it would only be healthy in its purest, unadulterated form. Just like human breast milk is. But we sure as hell don't consume cows' milk in its purest, unadulterated form. Nowadays, cows are injected with bovine growth hormone (BGH). (BGH milk is also referred to as rBGH—recombinant Bovine Growth Hormone or GE—genetically engineered.) Fifty years ago, the average milk production rate of a cow was 2,000 pounds a year. Today, the top producers provide up to 50,000 pounds a year![140] This is far from natural. (Imagine if your wife just gave birth and was injected with some crazy-ass hormone that made her boobs produce *twenty-five* times more milk than they would on their own.)

Dr. Samuel Epstein, professor emeritus of Environmental and Occupational Medicine at the School of Public Health at the University of Illinois at Chicago, has authored or coauthored thirteen books, published nearly three hundred peer-reviewed scientific articles, and is the leading international expert on BGH. He's also an internationally recognized authority on the mechanisms of carcino-

The Dairy Disaster

genesis, the causes and prevention of cancer, and the toxic and carcinogenic effects of environmental pollutants. (And he has, like, a million letters after his name: MD, DPath., DTM&H.) Dr. Epstein literally wrote "the book" on BGH: *What's in Your Milk?*[141] The beginning of his BGH journey started with a phone call he received from an angry farmer in 1989. The farmer was involved in the secret testing trials for BGH, and he wanted any scientific information available on the hormone. When Dr. Epstein admitted a lack of knowledge about the hormone, the farmer responded angrily to the effect of, "If it makes my cows sick, their milk will also make people sick. So it's damn well your job to find out." So Dr. Epstein began his inquiry. Six months later, he received a package that was sent anonymously. Its contents appeared to be records stolen directly from the FDA files—confidential data from BGH trials. And they included information that had been previously undisclosed, revealing a wide range of serious veterinary dangers associated with BGH.[142] You shouldn't be surprised to learn that the shit surrounding BGH is every bit as shady as aspartame's. Especially because Monsanto, the same company that owned NutraSweet, is the giant behind BGH. (BGH is sold to farmers under the trade name POSILAC.)[143] Dr. Epstein sent copies of the incriminating documents to Congressman John Conyers, who publicly stated, "Monsanto and the FDA have chosen to suppress and manipulate animal health test data . . . in efforts to approve commercial use of rBGH."[144]

Both Monsanto and the FDA knowingly and falsely claimed that:

* **There is no difference between milk from BGH cows and untreated cows.**

Um, bullshit. According to Dr. Epstein, "GE milk is entirely different from natural milk: nutritionally, biochemically, pharmacologically, and immunologically."[145]

* **BGH is harmless to cows.**[146]

Um, bullshit again. Its own package insert lists sixteen harmful health effects![147] And studies showed that cows treated with BGH had chronic inflammation of internal organs, ulcerating injection site reactions, and deep carcass damage. Almost half the injected cows became infertile! And the majority suffered from anemia and chronic mastitis—a bacterial infection resulting from inflamed udders. So what does all this mean? Cows injected with BGH are also treated with antibiotics and other drugs, many unapproved and illegal. During a single lactation period, one cow received 120 drug treatments![148] All lactating mammals excrete toxins through their milk, including hormones, antibiotics, pesticides, and chemicals.[149] So when you consume dairy products from cows treated with BGH, you're ingesting all that shit, too! By the way, remember, approximately *70 percent* of all the antibiotics made in the United States each year are administered to farm animals, causing antibiotic resistance in humans.[150]

* **BGH milk is safe for human consumption.**

Triple dose of bullshit! BGH milk has high levels of Insulin Growth Factor (IGF-1), which has been consistently linked to breast, colon, and prostate cancers.[151]

You should be so worked up right now that you're almost spitting blood. We're all being killed slowly so people can shove fistfuls of green fucking paper in their greedy-ass pockets. BGH milk is banned in Australia, New Zealand,[152] all of the European Union, Canada, Japan, and every other industrialized country in the world. Both the World Trade Organization and the United Nations Food Standards Body refuse to endorse the hormone's safety.[153] But BGH is legal here, in the United States. It's so baffling that we're supposed to be one of the most advanced nations in the world.

Pus, Chemicals, or Both?

Got pus? In factory farms, there is no gentle farmer milking cows with a bucket between his feet. Clamps are attached to cows' udders and cows are milked by machine. (Ask your wife how she'd like having clamps attached to her boobs immediately after giving birth.) The udders become sore and infected. Pus forms. But the machines keep on milking, sucking the dead white blood cells into the milk. In the good ol' U.S. of A., we have the highest allowable upper limit of pus concentration in the world—almost double the international standard.[154] Instead of saying, "It's as American as apple pie," we can start saying, "It's as American as pus in your milk!" Yeehaw!

Oh yeah, we're not done yet. To get rid of all the pus, bacteria, and other grossness, milk has to be pasteurized. (Meaning, they gotta boil the hell out of it.) So even if cows' milk were good for humans—it isn't—this process destroys beneficial enzymes, makes calcium less available, and creates radioactive particles.[155]

Pus and radioactive particles aren't the only dangers lurking in your milk. Oh no, batting third is dioxin, a known human carcinogen.[156] Dioxins are unintentional by-products from industrial practices (like chemical manufacturing, metal refining, combustion, etc.). They get

The Dairy Disaster

released into the air and then they settle into water (affecting the fish) and onto grasslands (affecting the cattle that graze there). Dioxin gets readily absorbed into the flesh of the animals exposed to it. So when we eat the animals' flesh or consume the milk of the animals, we get exposed to dioxin.[157]

PCBs are other sinister chemicals that accumulate in fat. Even though PCBs have been banned in the United States for more than twenty years, they still persist in our environment and will continue to contaminate our meat and dairy for many years.[158]

We're still going. Brominated flame retardants (BFRs) resemble PCBs chemically. Research suggests that BFRs have adverse affects on the brain, liver, and reproductive system, and on thyroid function. Where do these BFR bad boys accumulate? Animal-based foods.[159] A more specific class of BFRs is polybrominated diphenyl ethers (PBDEs). It's suggested that PBDE exposure in the United States is among the highest in the world. Flame retardants used in household items pollute our environment. Farm animals and fish absorb these pollutants. When we eat their flesh or drink their milk, we're exposed.[160]

Dirty Secrets, Leukemia, and a Whole Lot of Drama

Wish we were done, but we need to talk about Johne's disease. Oh, wait, you've never heard of it? Of course you haven't. Because Johne's (pronounced yo-Neez) disease is "something that farmers talk about secretly—whisper behind hands."[161] One dairy scientist calls it the "whispering campaign," and stated he had never heard a frank, open discussion about it.[162] One dairy farmer referred to Johne's as "a dirty word. It's like AIDS—you don't talk about it."[163] When the USDA released a report on 2,500 dairy producers in 1997, they estimated that up to 40 percent of those dairy herds were infected. (They also conceded that it was likely an *underestimate*.)[164] Health experts correlate the high rate of Johne's disease in cattle with the growing epidemic of Crohn's disease in humans.[165] How is it transmitted? People suffering from Crohn's disease suffer from uncontrollable diarrhea. And apparently, cows with Johne's disease suffer the same affliction. (Get your barf bag handy.) The diarrhea can come shooting out of the cow in liquid form. And because her butt is so close to her udders, poo gets on her udders. And unless someone takes the time to wash and clean the udders of every cow before every milking, the infected fecal matter

The Dairy Disaster

makes its way into the milk.[166] Bonus: Within that poo, there can be as many as one trillion paratuberculosis bugs per gram.[167] Surprise, surprise: The good ol' U.S. of A. has the highest incidence of Crohn's disease in the world.[168] Hey, instead of, "It's as American as pus in your milk," it can be, "It's as American as poopy milk and Crohn's disease."

Unless we want to change it to, "It's as American as leukemia." The bovine leukemia virus involves about 80 percent of dairy herds![169] The virus can be killed *if* the milk is pasteurized and pasteurized correctly. But sometimes milk is sold "raw." In a study of randomly collected raw samples, the virus was detected in *two thirds*![170] Now you're probably thinking, "Oh, phew. I don't buy raw milk products." But what if the milk you do buy isn't pasteurized correctly? Or what if the milk processing plant has an accidental "cross contamination" between raw and pasteurized milk? Not surprisingly, states with known leukemic dairy herds have higher rates of human leukemia.[171]

Yes, we are saying many scientists in the medical research field know that dairy is bad for you. Yes, we are saying many executives in the dairy industry are well aware of this fact but make claims that milk "does a body good." How do they get away with this? Easily. They spend hundreds of millions of dollars every year to market their products. And average consumers don't spend their time perusing medical journals, but they do read magazines and watch television.

What about medical doctors? Why do they believe that milk is beneficial? It is a sad fact that in this country, most doctors know almost nothing about nutrition. Remember, doctors receive very little nutritional training in medical school.[172] They have been duped like the rest of us.

But don't the government and U.S. Department of Agriculture protect us from all this? Hell no. Sickeningly high levels of pesticides found in dairy meet government standards. Records from the Food and Drug Administration show that "virtually 100 percent of the cheese products produced and sold in the United States has detectable pesticide residues."[173]

By the way, don't think you can worm your way out of the dairy drama by eating "low-fat" dairy products. They're still made from cows' milk, so they're just as pus-y, grody, and contaminated. Not to mention they can have a relative overburden of protein and lactose. Too much protein can tax the kidneys and leach calcium from the bones.[174] And undigested lactose encourages the growth of bacteria in our intestines.[175] Gross.

Organic Dairy Sucks

Sorry, but organic dairy products aren't much better. You've let the dairy industry dupe you long enough. Don't dupe yourself. Don't allow your addiction to cheese or your outdated beliefs con you that organic dairy is some clean, pure, magical entity. These products *may* be free of the chemical pesticides, hormones, and antibiotics, but they too can have fecal matter and pus. And in case you forgot everything you just read in this chapter: The consumption of dairy has been linked to heart disease; diabetes; obesity; osteoporosis; kidney stones; cataracts; macular degeneration; multiple sclerosis; Alzheimer's; and prostate, colon, rectal,[176] and breast cancer.[177] Use your head! Cow's milk is for baby cows; it is not good for humans! (Even if it were, how would you like it if right after your wife gave birth someone snatched your baby away, stuck him in a veal crate, attached clamps to your wife's nipples, milked her, and then sold the milk for profit? The fact that they are "just" cows doesn't make it any less cruel or sadistic.)

It's all too unbelievable, right? We know. But bear in mind, we have nothing to gain by telling you all this. In fact, we've got everything to lose. The billion-dollar dairy industry is so rich and powerful, they could sue us for everything we have. (Remember when the cattle ranchers sued Oprah, unsuccessfully, for publicly disparaging beef?) It would cost them next to nothing, but the legal fees alone would bankrupt us in minutes. We're risking our own livelihoods to tell you this. So don't be skeptical of us, like we're trying to sell you the Brooklyn Bridge. You've already bought the book, so whether you believe us or not doesn't add any money to our coffers. We're telling you this, and hoping you'll believe it, because it's true. And because we can't bear that *anyone* would eat or drink this poison!

Um, What's the Point of Milk, Again?

Okay, so you know you don't need milk for calcium, but what about vitamin D? Well, milk can't be trusted for that, either! According to PCRM, "Samplings of milk have found a significant variation of vitamin D content, with some samplings having had as much as 500 times the indicated level, while others had little or none at all." FYI: Too much vitamin D can be toxic![178] But it's been reported that "vitamin D is routinely added to milk 'above and beyond' the legal requirements."[179] Don't get us wrong—vitamin D is important. It aids in calcium and phosphorous absorption. But you don't need to

The Dairy Disaster

play Russian roulette with cows' milk to get it. Just get off your ass, open your door, and go outside. The body makes vitamin D when the skin is exposed to the sun! How cool is that? (Depending on your skin tone and locale, you just need five to twenty minutes of sun a day, two to seven days a week, on your face and hands.)[180] However, be advised that many people don't get enough sunlight due to their lifestyles. And that sunscreen that protects against skin cancer also blocks the rays needed to make vitamin D. So be sure to eat vitamin D-fortified foods, like cereals, rice- and soymilks, or talk to your doctor about popping a vegan vitamin D supplement (go to your local health food store or visit vegetarianvitamin.com or veganessentials.com).

Milk is not a reliable source of minerals, either. You get much higher levels of manganese, chromium, selenium, and magnesium from fruits and vegetables. Fruits and veggies are also high in boron, which helps lessen the loss of calcium through urine. Consuming high amounts of dairy blocks iron absorption, contributing to iron deficiency.[181] Just eat a variety of colorful fruits and veggies and snack on raw nuts and seeds every day. Minerals are more absorbable from these sources than from milk.[182]

Yes, milk is high in calcium, but the calcium is not as absorbable as it is in plant foods. Note the calcium absorbability of the following foods, according to the *American Journal of Clinical Nutrition:*

> **Brussels sprouts** . . . 63.8 percent
> **Broccoli** . . . . 52.6 percent
> **Kale** . . . . 50 percent
> **Cow's milk** . . . . 2 percent[183]

Calcium is naturally abundant in and most readily absorbed from leafy greens (kale, mustard greens, collard greens, turnip greens, Swiss chard), bok choy, cabbage, broccoli, Brussels sprouts, okra, watercress, legumes, chickpeas, red beans, soybeans, almonds, sesame seeds, and sea vegetables (like seaweed). It can also be easily attained from fortified orange juice, apple juice, soymilk, rice milk, cereal, and calcium-processed tofu. And these foods don't come laden with fat, cholesterol, and a harmful excess of protein. These foods are nothing but good for ya. (Also, FYI, cows' milk is allowed to have *80* friggin' antibiotics in it![184] *Eighty!* Fortified juices and rice- or soymilks have zero antibiotics. You do the math.)

While we're all running around thinking cows' milk is the end-all, be-all for health, globally, we're among the minority. Worldwide, 65 percent of adults abstain from milk.[185] It's estimated that men under

The Dairy Disaster

fifty should aim for 1,000 milligrams of calcium per day and that men over fifty get 1,200 milligrams.[186] But don't think you can eat crap all day and then just pop a calcium supplement to make up for it. There's no substitute for healthy, calcium-rich foods. So take your viteys, if instructed, but eat well, too. Have five to eight servings per day of calcium-rich foods. And make sure you exercise—lazy-asses lose the calcium from their bones while active people retain theirs.[187] And quit fucking smoking already! It increases your risk for fractures[188] (and guarantees a foul-ass smelling mouth). P. S. Alcohol and steroids can also have a negative effect on bones.[189]

You will shit yourself when you see how much weight you lose from giving up dairy. The fat in the cheese is what gives it the taste and texture we love. Of the calories found in cheese, 70 to 80 percent come from fat. Even if you're buying the low-fat, part-skim bullshit, more than half the calories come from fat.[190] Fat-free? Give us a friggin' break! Remember what milk is for. It is designed to fatten baby cows. Do you really believe it can be altered into a fat-free, healthy, natural product? Get your head out of your ass. Milk = fat. Butter = fat. Cheese = fat. People who think these products can be natural and low-fat or fat-free = duped.

Now, if you're anything like us, eating gives you more joy than everything—yep, even sex. So you might be wondering, "What the hell am I gonna eat now that I know dairy is bad for me? I know how to get calcium, but how about pleasure?" Don't worry. We're on it. First off, soymilk, rice milk, and almond milk are great replacements for cows' milk. Just read the ingredients and make sure the one you buy is fortified or enriched (that means they added calcium and other good stuff). Also, avoid brands that have any form of sweeteners in the "milk." If you're trying to limit your sugar intake, you sure as hell don't want to waste your ration on friggin' rice milk. Next, get yourself some soy "butter." It tastes like the real deal and can be used just like butter—on toast, pancakes, even in recipes. Mmm! We could eat it with a spoon! Speaking of. . . . Have you tried soy ice cream or coconut milk ice cream? Seriously, it'll rock your world. Yes, you should be limiting your sugar intake, but if you *have* to have ice cream, rock the dairy-free. It is ridiculously good. Tofutti makes pretty decent dairy-free versions of cream cheese and sour cream. (Just be sure to read the ingredients and get the ones *without* hydrogenated oil.) And the best dairy-free cheeses on the market are Follow Your Heart and Teese. Feel free to try other brands, but read the

The Dairy Disaster

ingredients. The majority of soy cheeses on the market *aren't* dairy-free. Some contain casein, which is the milk protein that promotes all three stages of cancer growth, remember? Others contain whey. Uck. But Follow Your Heart and Teese receive our stamp of approval. If you're like most people, you've been buying the same crappy products for years. So be patient: it'll take a little time to locate all the dairy-free products, and it'll require trial and error to figure out which ones you like.

How about eggs? You know how when a woman is pregnant and she drinks alcohol or does drugs, it affects her unborn child? Well, it is the same with chickens and their unhatched eggs. When you eat eggs, you are ingesting all the same hormones, pesticides, chemicals, and steroids as if you were eating the chicken directly. So if you really believe that eating "just egg whites" isn't fattening, we've got a bridge we can sell ya. Eggs are high in saturated fat and are completely disgusting when you think about what you are eating. Try that for once—actually think about what you are eating. (FYI: Eggs are a hen's menstrual cycle. N-a-s-t-y.) Also, a new study of 57,000 people linked egg consumption with type 2 diabetes,[191] and another with increased risk of heart failure.[192] An Argentine study found that people who ate about one and a half eggs per week had almost *five* times the risk of colorectal cancer as those who ate less than eleven eggs a year.[193] After analyzing data from thirty-four different countries, the World Health Organization correlated egg consumption with colon and rectal cancer mortality.[194] Another study found that moderate egg consumption *tripled* the risk of developing bladder cancer.[195] So save your, "But what about organic, free-range eggs?" bullshit for someone else—someone who doesn't care about your colon, rectum, and bladder. Egg Beaters are made of real eggs, so they're a gross no-no. But if you take a slice of some firm or extra-firm tofu and press out the excess water, heat it up in a pan, and add a little soy butter, salt, pepper, and ketchup, you've got yourself a "fried egg." There's also an egg substitute in powder form for cooking and baking called Ener-G egg replacer. And many markets sell a pretty good tofu "egg" salad.

As the demand grows for good animal-free and dairy-free products, more companies will supply us with these foods. So let your consumer dollars voice your desire, and your body will be rewarded. If you can't find good stuff at your local store, venture out to the nearest health food store or Whole Foods. Or, flap your big gums and ask your store's manager to order the stuff for you. They'll usually accom-

The Dairy Disaster

modate special requests.

So yeah, we just told you that eggs and dairy products suck. Don't freak out. Going against the grain can feel uncomfortable, wrong, and totally fucking weird. After all, every doctor you've ever known has endorsed milk's safety and nutritional value. Unfortunately, they simply don't know any better. But bear in mind, there are many, many, many health experts, scientists, researchers, and doctors that vehemently oppose the claims of the dairy industry. Their voices are just drowned out by the billion-dollar industry. If what we've said in this chapter kinda rings true for you, but you still feel uncomfortable, do your own research. Take matters into your own hands. Collecting information can be the ultimate reassurance. It's disquieting to believe what others say, but when you've seen the proof yourself, it's a whole, new ballgame.

Chapter 6

You Are What You Eat

Now would be a good time to reflect on the adage, "You are what you eat." This statement, in all its simplicity, is brilliant. You are what you eat. You are a human body comprised of organs, blood and guts, and other shit. The food you put into your body works its way through your organs and bloodstream and is actually part of who you are. So every time you put crap in your body, you are crap.

Even knowing how abysmal the living conditions are for animals on factory farms, you cannot begin to imagine what the slaughter practices are like. "Humane" protocol calls for animals to be "stunned" before they are slaughtered. For cows, this means getting a metal bolt shot into the skull and then retracted. When done properly, using working equipment, this renders the cow unconscious. But time is money, and slaughterhouses operate at lightning speeds, some

You Are What You Eat

killing one animal every three seconds. Because thousands of frightened, struggling cows are not easy to stun, it is extremely common for a "stunner" to miss his mark.[196] Panicked hogs, also difficult to "hit," are stunned with an electric device. And if the jolt is too high, it bruises and bloodies the hogs' flesh (bad for business). Because business comes first on factory farms, the jolt is lowered, despite the fact that it doesn't properly stun the hogs.[197]

Stunned or not, cows and hogs are then "strung up" from the ceiling by a chain attached to their leg(s).[198] In theory, while they dangle there, they are supposed to be unconscious. But often they are fully conscious, struggling, screaming, and fearfully staring at the workers while they have their throats stabbed open.[199] Next, they travel along a "bleed rail," where they should bleed to death. But again, these large, frightened, struggling, conscious animals are difficult targets and the "stickers" (workers who cut their throats) don't always get a "good cut." Before cows can bleed to death, they are sent on their way to the "head-skinners," where the skin is sliced from their heads while they are still conscious.[200] Of course, this is excruciatingly painful, and the cows kick and struggle frantically. To avoid getting injured by the struggling animal, workers will sometimes sever the spinal cord with a knife blow to the back of the head. This paralyzes the animal below the neck so that the worker is safe. But these cows can still feel their skin being sliced away from their faces.[201] Next, their legs and head are chopped off, their entrails removed from their bodies, and then, finally, they are split in half. Often before hogs can bleed to death, they are dunked fully conscious into 140-degree scalding water to remove the hair from their bodies.[202]

Chickens, because they are so overcrowded and stressed, frequently peck each other, so their beaks are literally chopped off their faces. Even though chickens and turkeys comprise more than 98 percent of all land animals slaughtered for food, Congress exempted them from the Humane Slaughter Act, so there is no requirement to stun them.[203] But because it is easier to handle chickens that aren't fighting for their lives, their heads are dragged through a water bath that has been electrically charged. This paralyzes the birds, but does not stun them.[204] They are snatched up, shackled upside down, and their throats are slashed by machine at the rate of thousands per hour.[205] Next, they are dunked in scalding water to loosen their feathers. Again, they are supposed to be dead at this point, but if the machine misses its mark, or the chickens haven't bled to death, they are boiled alive. Then they are placed into a

You Are What You Eat

series of machines that literally beat their feathers off of them, still alive and having just been boiled.[206] All the while, they are being handled like rubber toys: grabbed by their necks, feet, or wings and thrown around. You get the idea.

In egg-laying factories, male baby chicks are completely useless to farmers because they don't produce eggs. So workers snatch up chicks speeding by on a conveyer belt, quickly glance at their undersides, and then toss the "useless" males into the garbage or into macerators—machines that chop, tear, and break them into tiny, little pieces. Yes. Literally. Millions of male baby chicks are shredded alive or simply thrown away as trash, left to languish.

In her book *Slaughterhouse*, Gail Eisnitz, chief investigator for the Humane Farming Association, interviewed dozens of slaughterhouse workers throughout the country. *Every single one* admitted to abusing animals or neglecting to report those who did.[207] The following are quotes from slaughterhouse workers taken from her book. (They are quite graphic and difficult to read, but we implore you to read each one. Don't be an asshole. You can endure reading it if animals have to endure suffering it.)

"I seen them take those stunners—they're about as long as a yard stick—and shove it up the hog's ass. They do it with cows, too. And in their ears, their eyes, down their throat. They'll be squealing, and they'll just shove it right down there."[208]

"Hogs get stressed out pretty easy. If you prod them too much they have heart attacks. If you get a hog in a chute that's had the shit prodded out of him and has a heart attack or refuses to move, you take a meat hook and hook it into his bunghole [anus]. You're dragging these hogs alive, and a lot of times the meat hook rips out of the bunghole. I've seen hams—thighs—completely ripped open. I've also seen intestines come out. If the hog collapses near the front of the chute, you shove the meat hook into his cheek and drag him forward."[209] "Or in their mouth. The roof of their mouth. And they're still alive."[210]

"Pigs on the kill floor have come up and nuzzled me like a puppy. Two minutes later I had to kill them—beat them to death with a pipe."[211]

"These hogs get up to the scalding tank, hit the water and start screaming and kicking. Sometimes they thrash so much they kick water out of the tank. . . . Sooner or later they drown. There's a rotating arm that pushes them under, no chance for them to get out. I'm not sure if they burn to death before they drown, but it takes them a couple of minutes to stop thrashing."[212]

"Sometimes I grab it [a hog] by the ear and stick it right through the eye. I'm not just taking its eye out, I'll go all the way to the hilt, right up through the brain, and wiggle the knife."[213]

"Only you don't just kill it, you go in hard, push hard, blow the windpipe, make it drown in its own blood. Split its nose. A live hog would be running around the pit. It would just be looking up at me and I'd be sticking, and I would just take my knife and—eerk—cut its eye out while it was just sitting there. And this hog would just scream."[214]

"I could tell you horror stories about cattle getting their heads stuck under the gate guards, and the only way you can get it out is to cut their heads off while they're still alive."[215]

"He'll kick them [hogs], fork them, use anything he can get his hands on. He's already broken three pitchforks so far this year, just jabbing them. He doesn't care if he hits its eyes, head, butt. He jabs them so hard he busts the wooden handles. And he clubs them over the back."[216]

"I've seen live animals shackled, hoisted, stuck, and skinned. Too many to count, too many to remember. It's just a process that's continually there. I've seen shackled beef looking around before they've been stuck. I've seen hogs (that are supposed to be lying down) on the bleeding conveyor get up after they've been stuck. I've seen hogs in the scalding tub trying to swim."[217]

"I seen guys take broomsticks and stick it up the cow's behind, screwing them with a broom."[218]

"I've drug cows till their bones start breaking, while they were still alive. Bringing them around the corner and they get stuck up in the doorway, just pull them till their hide be ripped, till the blood just drip on the steel and concrete. Breaking their legs. . . . And the cow be crying with its tongue stuck out. They pull him till his neck just pop."[219]

"One time I took my knife—it's sharp enough—and I sliced off the end of a hog's nose, just like a piece of bologna. The hog went crazy for a few seconds. Then it just sat there looking kind of stupid. So I took a handful of salt brine and ground it into his nose. Now that hog really went nuts, pushing its nose all over the place. I still had a bunch of salt left in my hand—I was wearing a rubber glove—and I stuck the salt right up the hog's ass. The poor hog didn't know whether to shit

You Are What You Eat

or go blind."[220]

"Nobody knows who's responsible for correcting animal abuse at the plant. The USDA does zilch."[221]

Eisnitz chronicled the constant failure of U.S. Department of Agriculture inspectors to stop this abuse and their willingness to look the other way. In addition, she exposed the USDA's blatant tolerance for allowing contaminated meat into the human food supply. Think about it. *Ten billion* land animals a year! Do you think the USDA has enough inspectors to supervise the humane and safe slaughter of *ten billion* animals a year? Of course the inspectors tolerate abuse and contaminated meat; they're overwhelmed, to say the least. Even if every single inspector did a good job (they don't), the factory workers can easily bypass the system. Eisnitz interviewed one worker from a horse slaughterhouse, who said, "Might be part of him's [a contaminated horse] bad, might be the pneumonia's traveled everywhere. I'd drag him back, and my boss would tell me to cut the hindquarters off and bring him into the cooler. The meat's supposed to be condemned, but still you'd cut it up and bag it." When Eisnitz asked, "But don't they have to be stamped 'USDA inspected'?" he responded, "He [his boss] got the stamper. He can stamp it himself when the doc leaves. . . . You take a condemned horse, skin him, cut him up, sell the meat. . . . We've sold it as beef."[222] According to one former Perdue worker, the poultry plants are filthy. She said there were flies, rats, and 5-inch long flying cockroaches covering the walls and floors.[223] Believe it or not, it gets worse: "After they are hung, sometimes the chickens fall off into the drain that runs down the middle of the line. This is where roaches, intestines, diseased parts, fecal contamination, and blood are washed down. Workers [vomit] into the drain. . . . Employees are constantly chewing and spitting out snuff and tobacco on the floor. . . Sometimes they have to relieve themselves on the floor. . . . The Perdue supervisors told us to take the fallen chickens out of the drain and send them down the line."[224] A USDA inspector said of the cockroaches, "One time we shined a flashlight into a hole they were crawling in and out, and they were so thick it was like maggots, you couldn't even see the surface."[225] A worker at another poultry plant said, "Every day, I saw black chicken, green chicken, chicken that stank, and chicken with feces on it. Chicken like this is supposed to be thrown away, but instead it would be sent down the line to be processed."[226] Another worker at another plant said, "I personally have seen rotten meat—

you can tell by the odor. This rotten meat is mixed with the fresh meat and sold for baby food. We are asked to mix it with the fresh food, and this is the way it is sold. You can see the worms inside the meat."[227] No comment. We are simply speechless.

Animals are intelligent, emotional, social creatures. Researchers at Bristol University in Britain discovered that cows actually nurture friendships and bear grudges. One study showed cows displaying excitement while solving intellectual challenges.[228]

Chickens are as smart as mammals, including some primates, according to research done by animal behaviorist Dr. Chris Evans of Macquarie University in Australia. They are apt pupils and can learn by watching the mistakes of others. One researcher conducted a study that demonstrated chickens' ability to use switches and levers to change the temperature of their surroundings. A PBS documentary revealed chickens' love for television and music.[229] And Discovery reported recently, "Chickens do not just live in the present, but can anticipate the future and demonstrate self-control, something previously attributed only to humans and other primates."[230]

Pigs can play video games! They've been labeled as more intelligent than dogs and three-year-old humans. They too can indicate their temperature preferences.[231]

Even fish have feelings. Dr. Donald Broom, scientific adviser to the British government, explains, "The scientific literature is quite clear. Anatomically, physiologically and biologically, the pain system in fish is virtually the same as in birds and animals." Fish, like "higher vertebrates," have neurotransmitters similar to endorphins that relieve suffering. Of course, the only reason for their nervous systems to produce painkillers is to relieve pain.[232]

For some lame-ass reason, there's this bullshit notion that men who eat meat, or ride bulls, or hunt and fish are "manly." We've even seen redneck bumper stickers claiming, "Real men eat meat." Sorry, but there's nothing manly about contributing to the torture and slaughter of innocent animals. It's actually selfish, scary, and barbaric.

Animals hear the screaming and crying of other animals being slaughtered and are terrified. They know they are about to be killed, and they are panic-stricken. When their young are taken from them, cows kick stall walls in rage and frustration and literally cry with grief. Think of how you feel when you are angry, afraid, and grief-stricken. Bear in mind the physical feelings that accompany these emotions. These emotions—fear, grief, and rage—produce chemical changes in our bodies. They do the same to animals. Their blood pressures rise. Adrenaline courses through their bodies. You are eating high blood pressure, stress, and adrenaline. You are eating fear, grief, and rage. You are eating suffering, horror, and murder. You are eating cruelty. Real men eat meat?

Although a minuscule percentage of meat in the United States comes from free-range farms, how do you even know it is really free-range? Companies want us to believe that products labeled "free-range" or "free-roaming" are derived from animals who spent their short lives outdoors, enjoying sunshine, fresh air, and the company of other animals. But labels other than "organic" on egg cartons are not subject to any government regulations. In addition, the USDA doesn't regulate "free-range" or "free-roaming" claims for beef products.[233] Because there are no agencies governing these claims, do you take the word of someone who makes a living on blood money? And even if the farm was truly free-range and humane, the animals are still being sent to horrific slaughterhouses. (An undercover video of a kosher slaughterhouse revealed animals suffering the worst abuse and torture. Check it out at HumaneKosher.com.)[234] Many animals don't even survive the transport from their factory- or free-range farm to slaughter. Up until very recently, the only law in existence dictating care for transported animals was related to *train* transport. But it just so happens that 95 percent of animals are transported by *truck*.[235] It's difficult to believe the new guidelines are being complied with or enforced. Animals receive little to no food or water or protection from the elements. Millions of animals are dead on arrival or too injured or sick to move. They don't get to stop for bathroom breaks, so the animals are forced to stand in their own urine and feces. In the wintertime, the animals' flesh and feet will actually freeze to the bottom and sides of the truck. So upon arrival, they are literally ripped away from the truck. One worker interviewed by Eisnitz said, "They freeze to that steel railing. They're still alive, and they'll hook a cable on it and pull it out, maybe pull a leg off."[236]

Assuming you started with a healthy animal (highly unlikely), you've now eaten hormones, pesticides, steroids, antibiotics, fear, grief, and rage. You are what you eat. But what if the animal wasn't healthy? Animals that are too sick or injured to walk are literally dragged to slaughter—either by forklift, or by chaining the animal to a truck. The USDA still allowed these animals, referred to as "downers," to be slaughtered for human consumption[237] despite the growing

You Are What You Eat

number of mad cow disease cases (a deadly and incurable disease that can be transmitted to humans through the consumption of cow flesh). Consumer and animal rights groups have been lobbying to keep downers out of the food chain for more than a decade—to no avail. Thankfully, in 2009, almost immediately into his presidency, Barack Obama announced that downed cows could no longer be part of the food supply. Hopefully, the ban will be complied with and enforced. If it isn't, in addition to all the other filth you're eating, you're also eating whatever illness the animal has. Bear in mind, downed pigs, goats, sheep, chickens, and turkeys can still be killed for human consumption. Cruel and gross. Real men eat meat?

Let's make believe that all the animals killed for human consumption are healthy, happy, free of antibiotics, steroids, and pesticides and are humanely raised and slaughtered. Pretend you are eating "perfect meat." Great. But what exactly are you eating? Have you thought about this even once in the last decade, or ever? "Meat" is the decomposing, decaying, rotting flesh of a dead animal. As soon as an animal dies, it starts "breaking down." How long has passed between when the animal was slaughtered and the time you are eating it? It could be weeks, even months. You want to put a dead animal corpse— that has been rotting away for months—in your mouth? In your body? Because meat is muscle tissue, it oxidizes in an open environment and turns brown. So most meat markets will scrape off the brown parts to make it look more appealing. Another trick of the trade is using tinted lighting in open meat cases to enhance the meat's color.[238] Restaurants and ranchers might call their meat "aged to perfection," but no matter how you slice it, it's still a putrefying corpse. Real men eat meat?

Just because you can't see what's happening doesn't mean it doesn't exist. Every time you have a craving for meat or dairy, remember what goes on inside every slaughterhouse, processing plant, and grocery store. Linda McCartney said it best: "If slaughterhouses had glass walls, we'd all be vegetarians."[239] For added motivation with your new diet, visit GoVeg.com and order a free vegetarian starter kit.

So now you are officially vegan, a person who doesn't eat *any* animal products. No meat, chicken, pork, fish, eggs, milk, cheese, or butter. Not only are you a real man, but you're hotter than fucking ever. Seriously. There's nothing hotter than a man who is a) compassionate, b) selfless, and c) secure enough with his manhood that he doesn't need to eat animal products to prove he's packing heat. Yes, it can be challenging to avoid animal products, but you will reap the karmic rewards of being vegan. For starters, the ratio of vegan women to vegan men is about a million to one, so you'll have your pick of the litter. But more important, you're sparing the lives of approximately one hundred animals a year.[240]

And every environmentalist knows that factory farming is completely destroying the environment. As ridiculous as it sounds, the methane resulting from the burps and farts of cows and pigs is directly responsible for global warming.[241] The nitrous oxide resulting from the manure decomposition of ten billion farm animals a year is another major contributor.[242] And all the carbon dioxide caused by the production of meat and dairy is yet another factor. Believe it or not, according to the United Nations Food and Agriculture Organization, raising animals for food causes significantly more greenhouse gas emissions than cars[243]—about forty percent more![244] This warrants repeating: raising animals for food causes forty percent more greenhouse gas emissions than cars. So you'd do more good for the planet switching from a meat-based diet to a plant-based diet than from trading in your Hummer for a Prius. (While that's true, it's gotta be said: Hummers are for dicks. Think about it.) According to the

United Nations' 400-page report, eating meat is the number one human cause of global warming, "one of the top two or three most significant contributors to the most serious environmental problems, at every scale from local to global," and causes "problems of land degradation, climate change and air pollution, water shortage and water pollution, and loss of biodiversity."[245] According to the Environmental Protection Agency, factory farms are the largest polluters of U.S. waterways.[246] Try to imagine, if you even can, the sheer volume of shit and piss of ten billion farm animals, every year, in the United States alone. It's horrifying. Think about how much land, food, water, and energy it takes just to grow food for these farm animals. Now think about how many resources it takes to transport this food to the animals. Now think about how much land, water, and energy it takes to raise these animals. Now get this: The amount of land, food, water, and energy used to raise ten billion animals a year for slaughter could be used to grow food for *all of the starving people in the world*. The United Nations called the diversion of crops to be turned into biofuels "a crime against humanity."[247] Agreed—100 million tons of crops that go to cars instead of starving people is wrong, wrong, wrong.[248] But what about the more than 750 million

You Are What You Eat

tons of corn and wheat that go to feed farm animals?[249] Or the 80 percent of the global soy crop that is also fed to them and not people?[250] Wrong on so many levels. Please, don't just skip ahead without fully grasping this: your being vegan is actually a step toward ending world hunger. Really.

So you shouldn't eat cows, chickens, pigs, fish, milk, cheese, or eggs. So what the hell should you eat? Pretty much everything else: fruits, vegetables, legumes, nuts, seeds, and whole grains. Deep down, you've known all along that these foods are best for you; now it's time to get back on track. Our diets have strayed so far off course from where they belong; we've allowed meat to take center stage, with grains and vegetables playing supporting roles. Wrong, wrong, wrong. There is a plethora of great-tasting, healthy, wholesome foods that you've likely been neglecting for years. Well, those days are over. Get back to the basics and enjoy all these excellent foods you forgot about. And enjoy all the health benefits they offer.

Can you remember back to your grade-school days when you learned about photosynthesis? Plants store the sun's energy, which we receive by eating them. If you can, just picture the light energy from the sun beaming down to the vegetables and fruits, and as we eat those foods, imagine that energy being transmitted into our bodies. Our nervous systems are maintained and stimulated by this light. What an amazing gift from nature—to be able to eat such pure foods that give our bodies so much!

However, be advised, all fruits and vegetables are not created equal. Plants need vitamins and minerals to function and grow properly. When they are sprayed with pesticides and grown in chemically treated soil, they won't absorb all the proper nutrients. This results in a loss of enzymes. So, organic fruits and vegetables—ones that have been grown in pure, untreated soil and without pesticides—have far more enzymes than their conventionally grown counterparts.[251]

Any scientist can tell you that food has an "energy" or "life" to it. Anyone with common sense can tell you that eating a live, fresh fruit is healthier than eating a cooked, canned, preserved one. Why? Because this "life" comes from the plant's energy, nutrients, phytochemicals, and enzymes. Enzymes are living biochemical factors that we need to survive. They are critical for digestion, breathing, reproduction, and the functioning of DNA and RNA. They also help repair and heal our organs, detoxify our bodies, carry out our nerve impulses, and help us think.

You Are What You Eat

There are three types of enzymes: metabolic, digestive, and food. Fortunately, we produce our own metabolic enzymes, which run the whole body, maintain our health, and defend us from illness and infection. But our own enzyme supplies are limited. So to continue healthy bodily functions, we need to supplement with food. When we eat, our bodies release digestive enzymes to break down the food. If we eat foods devoid of enzymes, such as meat, processed food, and even just overcooked food (high temperatures destroy enzymes), our bodies have to work much harder.[252] Harder work means using more of our precious enzymes. Over time, this can result in an enlargement of the digestive organs and the endocrine glands. (Studies have shown that the increased weight of these organs accompanies obesity.)[253] This lack of enzymes can also cause a disruption in the body's ability to make enough metabolic enzymes. But when we eat foods high in enzymes, such as fruits, salad, or lightly steamed veggies, we get an enzyme boost along with the meal, so our bodies don't have to work so hard. There is no greater defender of our bodies than enzymes. When not in use for digestion, enzymes are busy repairing and cleaning our bodies.[254] So don't go throwing your enzymes away on shit!

So how do we get these enzymes into our bodies? We just need to make the following foods part of our daily diets: fruits (especially pineapples, papayas, bananas, and mangos), raw or lightly steamed vegetables, raw nuts and seeds, wheat grass, sea vegetables, garlic, and legumes. Juicing is a great way to detoxify your body and get a lot of enzymes, but you must drink it right away.[255] As soon as a fruit is peeled, or cut, or juiced, it begins to lose its enzymes.[256] So, buying a gallon of fresh-squeezed juice isn't as beneficial as making your own daily. Packaged juice has been pasteurized, and the heat destroys the enzymes. Granted, it's still better to drink pasteurized juice than soda. So if you can't juice for yourself, do the best you can.

Well, there you have it. Fruits and vegetables are the answer. And unless you are an idiot who wants cancer, obesity, and enlarged organs, organic is the way to go. You are what you eat. (And you're a real fucking man.)

Chapter 7

The Myths and Lies About Protein

With all the low-carb bullshit going on in this country, it's never been more necessary to establish the facts about protein. First and foremost, everyone seems to think that protein exists just to help build muscle—like protein is the big muscle-head at the gym. Yes, protein does form muscle tissue, but it has many more functions than that. Protein assures proper growth, maintenance, and repair of *all* body tissues (not just muscles). It also contributes to healing the body; production of blood cells, energy, and hormones; the formation of antibodies and hemoglobin; and the building of enzymes.[257] Those who don't get enough protein can suffer from decreased immunity, loss of muscle mass, improper growth, and weakening of the heart and respiratory system.[258]

So clearly, protein is an important part of any diet. But it shouldn't be the cornerstone of any diet, and this is where the high-protein/low-carb craze really misleads people. You know by now that complex carbs shouldn't be forsaken. But should you overload on protein? Hell, no. If we had a penny for every time some meathead asked us, "So where do you get your protein?" we'd be richer than Trump. Have you ever, in your entire life, heard of anyone in a developed country suffering from a protein deficiency? Did you ever see an elephant, moose, or giraffe jonesing for a protein fix? If you weren't blacked out on bourbon for the past four chapters, you should know by now: It is a complete urban myth that we need a massive amount of protein. Too much protein, especially animal protein, can impair our kidneys; leach calcium, zinc, B vitamins, iron, and magnesium from our bodies; and cause osteoporosis, heart disease, cancer, and obesity. In addition, high amounts of protein can damage our tissues, organs, and cells, contributing to faster aging.[259] Yikes! Know this: People in other cultures consume half the amount of protein that we do, yet they live longer, healthier lives.[260]

Although too much is harmful, protein is still vital to our health. Protein produces enzymes, hormones, neurotransmitters, and antibodies; replaces worn out cells; transports various substances throughout the body; and aids in growth and repair.[261] Basically, if you eat a well-balanced vegan diet, you'll get enough protein. But for all you annoying counters who want a stupid number to latch onto, here's a simple equation to find out how much protein you need:

Body weight (in pounds) x .36 = recommended protein intake[262]

(This number gives the average person

a large margin of safety.)[263]

Researchers at Harvard found that vegetarians (who don't live on junk food) get adequate amounts of protein in their diets.[264] The American Dietetic Association reports that eating a vegetarian diet provides twice the amount of protein needed daily.[265] In his book *Optimal Health*, Dr. Patrick Holford explains that "most people are in more danger of eating too much protein than too little."[266] So pick something else to be neurotic about (like your bald spot).

How do vegans get protein? Simply. We eat lentils, beans, peas, nuts, seeds, fruits, vegetables, whole-grains, and soy products (edamame, tofu, imitation cheeses and meats). When you eat well-balanced meals consisting of these foods, you are guaranteed to get sufficient protein. For example, for lunch, if you had a soy burger on a whole grain bun with avocado and tomato and a small side salad, you'd get 22 grams of protein. See how easy? If you want an extra boost, treat yourself to spirulina, high-protein algae that contains omega-3 and omega-6 fatty acids, B-12 (important for vegetarians), enzymes, and minerals. It also repairs free-radical damage (caused by chemicals that harm cells and contribute to premature aging, heart disease, and cancer), supports the immune system, fights cancer, and helps with hypoglycemia, anemia, ulcers, diabetes, and chronic fatigue syndrome. Spirulina also contains all nine essential amino acids.[267]

Amino acids, huh? Yep. There are twenty amino acids. Our bodies produce eleven, and the other nine essential amino acids can be obtained through food. Amino acids are the building blocks of protein. And yes, protein does build muscle. But even if you work out and want to build muscle, you don't need to overdose on animal protein (a ridiculous myth perpetuated by dumbbells). Bear in mind, some tough-ass motherfuckers are vegans or vegetarians: Tim VanOrden, a champion road-, mountain-, snowshoe-, and stair-climb racer;[268] John Salley, a four-time NBA champion; Brendan Brazier, an Ironman triathlete; Stan Price, world record holder for the bench

The Myths and Lies About Protein

press; Ridgely Abele, eight-time national karate champion; Peter Burwash, Davis Cup winner and professional tennis player; Peter Hussing, super heavy-weight boxing champion; Sixto Linares, world record holder of the 24-hour triathlon; Ben Matthews, U.S. Master's marathon champion; Dan Millman, world champion gymnast; Paavo Nurmi, long-distance runner winner and nine-time Olympic medalist and twenty-time world-record holder; Bill Pickering, world record-holding swimmer;[269] Sushil Kumar, Olympic bronze medalist wrestler;[270] Chris Campbell, Olympic wrestling champion; Keith Holmes, world-champion middleweight boxer; Bill Mannetti, power-lifting champion; Bill Pearl, four-time Mr. Universe; Andres Cahling, champion bodybuilder and Olympic gold medalist in the ski jump; Art Still, a Hall of Famer and MVP defensive end for the NFL;[271] Ricky Williams, NFL running back;[272] Ricardo Moreira, Ultimate Fighter;[273] Chris Price, Muay Thai and mixed martial arts fighter; Kenneth Williams, professional bodybuilder;[274] Jake Shields, mixed martial arts champion;[275] Jerry Stackhouse; NBA player;[276] Prince Fielder, MLB player; Tony Gonzalez, NFL player; Salim Stoudamire, NBA player; Desmond Howard, NFL player; Mac Danzig, UFC Champion; Pat Neshak, MLB player; Scott Jurek, ultramarathon champion;[277] Robert Cheeke, an International Natural Bodybuilding Association and International Natural Bodybuilding & Fitness Federation bodybuilder; Dave Scott, six-time Ironman winner; Murray Rose, Olympic swimmer with six medals; Al Oerter, four-time gold medalist discus thrower; Edwin Moses, two-time gold medalist hurdler; and Olympic star Carl Lewis, who said his best year on the track was the year he adopted a vegan diet.[278] Vegetarian athletes (and civilians) are constantly praising their plant-based diets for giving them more energy than they've ever had before.

So whether you're a professional athlete, or extremely active and look-ing to bulk up, or you're just the average Joe looking to meet your daily protein quota, where *should* this protein come from? Like any average American, your brain probably went back to the muscle-head at the gym, and you likely thought, "I need to get X grams of protein a day. I'll just eat more chicken, meat, or fish." (Notice we left dairy and eggs off that list. If you still want to consume eggs or dairy products after that last chap-ter, we're gonna kick your fat ass.) Somehow, we've all been conditioned into thinking (dairy, eggs), chicken, meat, and fish are the only foods in existence that have protein. However, this is simply not the case. And it's a good thing, because these foods present multiple health risks.

Just. Plain. Gross.

For starters, according to the USDA, 86 percent of all food poisoning is caused by animal foods.[279] There are all sorts of gross things you can get from eating meat, chicken, eggs, and fish (or from foods that touch these foods). You've all heard of salmonella, but how about campylobacter? Well, *Consumer Reports* tested store-bought broiler chickens nationwide and found salmonella and/or campylobacter contamination in nearly *half* of them, including those from organic, free-range, and kosher producers![280] You can also get salmonella from raw or undercooked eggs or products containing them. If you do get salmonella, be on the lookout for diarrhea, arthritis, colon damage, and the Grim Reaper.[281] E. coli is no picnic, either, and can be caught by ingesting raw dairy products or improperly cooked meat. Just so you know, the presence of E. coli is an indicator of fecal contamination. How'd you like a side of shit with those fries? A USDA study found detectable levels of E. coli in more than 99 percent of store-bought broiler chickens![282] Once infected, a person can expect bloody diarrhea and possibly even renal failure.[283] Oh, but don't worry. Processors spray chicken carcasses with disinfectant—inside and out.[284] (Gag! How'd you like a can of Lysol with those wings?)

Sex, Drugs, and Factory Farms

Well, even if we do get food poisoning, we can just take medicine, right? Hmm. Of the *ten billion* land animals slaughtered for food each year in America, almost all come from factory farms. Factory farms that raise cattle, pigs, chickens, egg-laying hens, veal calves, or dairy cows keep an enormous number of animals in a very small space. (For example, a chicken shed can have 30,000–50,000 chickens confined, each with less space than a standard sheet of paper.)[285] Egg-laying hens are crammed into cages so small they are unable to spread even one wing. Pigs and cows are kept in stalls so small they are unable to turn around or lie down. Broiler chickens are crowded so tightly into warehouse-type structures that they often peck or trample each other to death. Animals live in the filth of their own urine, feces, and vomit with infected, festering sores and wounds. To keep them alive in these unsanitary conditions, factory farmers give animals massive amounts of antibiotics.[286] But they don't sort through ten billion animals to see who's sick and might need it. They give it to all of them. Penicillin, tetracycline, and countless other antibiotics are routinely administered. When we eat the flesh of these animals, we're eating these antibiotics. This overuse of antibiotics leads to the development of new antibiotic-resistant bacterial strains.[287] Meaning, due to the abuse of antibiotics by factory farmers, new bacterial strains are forming (gross) and the antibiotics we'd normally take to combat them are rendered ineffective (scary). One USDA study found 67 percent of chicken and 66 percent of beef to be contaminated with "superbugs" that couldn't be killed by antibiotics.[288] Nasty. No wonder the European Union wants nothing to do with our meat. They only allow four antibiotics to be used on their livestock, none of which are used in human health care. Does Lady Liberty have any restrictions like these? Nope.[289] Our country allows farmers to feed the most toxic form of arsenic to broiler chickens.[290] You heard us. It's legal to feed arsenic to broiler chickens (to kill parasites and promote growth). Apparently, the USDA and FDA don't mind that researchers found arsenic residue in chicken at 100 percent of fast-food restaurants and 50 percent of supermarkets investigated.[291] Actually, there's arsenic in most American meat, but there's four times as much in chicken as in other meats.[292] Gnarly.

On factory farms, animals are raised in the smallest quarters possible where they're "grown" as large as possible to inflate the profit margin as much as possible. In addition to antibiotics and arsenic, anabolic steroids are routinely administered to the animals. It's been reported that approximately 99 percent of commercially raised cattle is treated with growth hormones![293] When we eat their flesh, we're eating the growth hormones. No wonder Americans are struggling with weight problems—we're ingesting growth hormones on a regular basis.

And no wonder reproductive cancers have skyrocketed since the 1950s—breast cancer has increased by 55 percent, testicular cancer has gone up by 120 percent, and prostate cancer has increased 190 percent![294] In addition to antibiotics and steroids, growth-promoting sex hormones are also given to farm animals routinely. For more than a decade, the FDA has allowed farmers to implant hormonal agents in the ears of cows. These include—but are in no way limited to—testosterone (male hormone), estradiol and progesterone (female hormones), and norgestomet (a synthetic progestin).[295] By the way, the estrogen estradiol is one of the most commonly used hormones for fattening cows. And it's a potent carcinogen.[296] S-c-a-r-y. Even scarier: A USDA survey of feedlots found that nearly half the cows had illegally misplaced implants in their muscle tissue, as opposed to their ears. (Let us add that the statistic represents the implants that were *visibly* misplaced.[297] The actual percentage could've been well above half.) These hormones can contribute to estrogen dominance, which, in women, has been linked to endometriosis; fibroids; and breast, ovarian, and cervical cancer. In men, estrogen dominance can cause prostate and testicular cancer, and even "male menopause." Don't laugh. Male menopause can include symptoms like impotence, testicular atrophy, breast growth, fatigue, depression, and reduction or loss of sex drive. Who's at the highest risk for male menopause? Those who worked on poultry farms, implanting chickens and turkeys with estrogen pellets![298] You do the math.

Mad Cow Disease, Chemicals . . . When Does It End?

Unfortunately, hormone use is not the only area the United States is lacking in regarding meat safety issues. In Japan, 100 percent of cattle slaughtered for human consumption is tested for mad cow disease.[299] Here, we test approximately .05714 percent.[300] (For those of you who are mathematically challenged, that's way less than one percent!) Former Agriculture Secretary Mike Johanns admitted that testing is not done to protect consumers from mad cow disease, but rather to discern the disease's prevalence.[301] How reassuring. Hmm, we wonder if that's why 65 nations have full or partial restrictions on importing our beef.[302] It could be that. Or it could be that the FDA approved the spraying of live viruses onto meat and poultry products (to combat listeria). Yeah, the spray contains six different viral strains, and meat companies aren't obligated to inform customers which products have been sprayed.[303]

Unfortunately, even if the USDA and FDA implemented bans on hormones, steroids, and antibiotics, our meat would still be contaminated with toxic chemicals. Here's how it works—Pesticides 101: Pesticides are used on crops to prevent bugs and weeds from destroying them. If it's a crop grown for us to eat, we wash them off, getting rid of some of the chemicals. If it's a crop used to feed *animals*, the pesticides are not washed off. And unlike crops grown for us to eat, crops grown for animals to eat have no limits on the amount of pesticides that can be used. More than 1.5 billion pounds of pesticides are used each year in this country![304] And approximately 80 percent are used on the four major animal-feed crops.[305] P. S. Pesticides are also sprayed directly onto the animals themselves to ward off parasites, insects, rodents, and fungi. So, you can see, the animals we're ingesting are subject to major pesticide ingestion and exposure for their

The Myths and Lies About Protein

entire lives. And when we ingest the animals, we're ingesting the pesticides, too. What you can't see is that the animals store these pesticides in their fat tissue and cells.[306] So when you eat meat, you're ingesting a higher amount of pesticides than you would if you ate the pesticide-treated food directly.

And unfortunately, pesticides aren't all we're getting. Herbicides, industrial wastes, PCBs, BFRs, BDFEs—they're polluting our waterways and affecting our food supply. But again, the fatty tissues of animals attract and concentrate these chemicals—"bio-accumulation." And as all these environmental pollutants move up the food chain, they're concentrated even more—"biomagnification."[307] So a corn crop may have a specific amount of toxic residue in it. Then a cow, chicken, or pig eats the corn and absorbs a larger amount of toxic residue. Then a human eats the cow, chicken, or pig and absorbs an even larger amount of toxic residue.

Just one of these chemicals on its own would be scary enough. But the abundance and complex interaction of so many can wreak havoc on the endocrine, hormonal, neurological, immunological, and reproductive systems.[308]

Something's Fishy

Sadly, our waters aren't any better; they too are alarmingly polluted. So eating fish (or other seafood) is just as dangerous as eating meat. Their flesh also accumulates and absorbs chemical pollutants, like mercury, organochlorides, PCBs, and others. It works like this: Chemical levels in water may be low enough to receive passing grades from the Environmental Protection Agency (EPA). But the chemical concentration in algae can increase by up to 250. When the zooplankton eats the algae, the concentration can double. When the tiny shrimp eat the zooplankton, the concentration can be 45,000 times higher. By the time the little fish eat the shrimp, and the big fish eat the little fish, and we eat the big fish, we're looking at a concentration 25 million times that which was found in the water![309]

Don't be thinking "farm-raised" fish are clean and pure. The feed given to farm-raised salmon has high levels of chemical pollutants, making them practically toxic in comparison with ocean-caught fish (which you now know are polluted).[310] Farmed salmon are fed artificial dyes to make them appear pink like wild salmon, instead of the unnatural, murky gray color they actually are.[311]

Yes, some fish contain beneficial omega-3 fatty acids, but you can get those from foods that aren't laden with heavy metals, toxins, saturated fat and cholesterol.[312] So even though omega-3s are heart-healthy, a recent study in the *British Medical Journal* reported that eating fish did *not* have a beneficial effect on heart health.[313] However, a study in the *American Journal of Cardiology* praised walnuts' positive effect on arteries[314]—unsurprising since walnuts are rich in omega-3s, cholesterol-free, and low in saturated fat.[315] (Other nuts, leafy greens, and flax seeds are also good sources of omega-3s.)

Friggin' Protein

Whether it's milk, cheese, eggs, chicken, pork, beef, or fish, animal foods are the only ones that have cholesterol. They also contain a less than ideal fat profile. And that's in addition to all the bacteria, hormones, steroids, pesticides, chemical pollutants, and antibiotics! Um, so why do we eat them—for protein? Yep, basically, we risk heart disease, obesity, diabetes, and all sorts of cancers because we've been brainwashed into thinking these are the only foods with protein. But you now know we can easily obtain adequate protein by eating a variety of fruits, vegetables, whole grains, nuts, seeds, and legumes. And it just so happens that those foods have a variety of health benefits, too! Again, eat all types of beans, peas, lentils, nuts, and seeds; breads and pastas made from whole grains; bulgur; millet; barley; quinoa; buckwheat; oats; amaranth; brown rice; potatoes; sweet potatoes; broccoli; kale; asparagus; avocados, soybeans; tofu —the list is endless, really. Fruits. Veggies. Legumes. Nuts. Seeds. Whole grains. All sources of protein.

And contrary to popular belief (surprise, surprise), meat is not the only "complete" protein. Meaning, soybeans also have all the amino acids our bodies can't produce on their own.[316] But even if you don't eat soy, you can get all the aminos by eating a variety of fruits, veggies, legumes, nuts, seeds, and whole grains. And it doesn't have to be in one sitting. As long as you're eating a variety of foods from those food groups, you're getting all the aminos you need![317]

Another common myth that has been debunked is the "food combining" theory. Animal flesh proteins are "complete," meaning they contain all nine essential amino acids in amounts similar to those found in human flesh. Plants have all these amino acids, too, just in slightly different amounts. It was previously believed that to create complete proteins from vegetarian foods, you needed to combine them in specific ways. For example, it was said rice and beans had to be eaten together to maximize their protein potential. However, it is now known that eating a variety of foods from plant sources provides all the building blocks we need. Further, the microorganisms and recycled cells in our intestinal tracts make complete proteins for us.[318] All we have to do is eat healthy, balanced diets.

The Soy Saga

Will soymilk give you man-boobs? Do men have wittle wee-wees because they eat tofu? There's so much madness surrounding soy, it's hard to know what the real "truth" is. Soy supporters claim it can do everything—lower cholesterol, reduce heart disease, and decrease risk of multiple cancers. Opponents claim it can depress thyroid function, cause cancer,[319] and negatively affect sperm.[320] Here's what we know to be "pro-soy true":

* Soybeans are "complete proteins," meaning they contain the essential amino acids our bodies don't manufacture.[321]

* Calorie for calorie, soybeans have twice as much protein as red meat and cheese, and ten times more protein than whole milk.[322]

* Soybeans are a good source of omega-3 fatty acids.[323]

* Soybeans have more iron, calcium, phosphorous, and B vitamins than eggs.[324]

* The majority of studies claiming soy has negative effects were conducted on animals. And animal tests are simply unreliable indicators, as the biology of each species varies greatly. (Cases in point: Thalidomide tested safe in animals, but caused horrendous birth defects in children. Diet phenom "fen-phen" tested safe in animals, but caused heart abnormalities in humans. Arthritis drug Opren tested safe in animals but killed humans!)[325]

* Entire civilizations have been eating soy for thousands of years without any ill effects and, in fact, have lower instances of cancer and heart disease.

  Here's what we know to be "anti-soy true":

* None of these civilizations have been eating as much soy as we eat now.

* None of these civilizations have been eating soy in so many highly processed forms. They've been eating tofu, tempeh, miso, and actual soybeans. Here and now, we have soy "meats," "cheeses," "ice creams," and even supplements. And soybean oil makes its way into a multitude of processed foods.

The Myths and Lies About Protein

* Soy is one of the most commonly genetically engineered crops around. So unless you're buying organic, you might be eating soybeans that have been genetically manipulated.

* Soy is one of the highest pesticide-yielding crops around. So unless you're buying organic, you might be getting a hefty dose of pesticides.

So what's all the drama about? Basically, it centers on isoflavones and phytoestrogens, chemical compounds found in soybeans (and other plant foods, too). Because isoflavones and phytoestrogens structurally resemble human estrogens, their safety has been questioned. However, anti-soy studies use an isolated, concentrated amount of soy isoflavones that exceed what a person would consume. And again, the studies showing negative effects are conducted on animals, who metabolize soy differently than we do. (Case in point: Humans can eat chocolate without incidence. However, chocolate can be fatal when ingested by dogs.)[326] In addition, when you extract certain components of many foods and test them in isolation, they can be harmful. But when eaten as part of whole foods in normal-sized servings, they are perfectly safe. Mushrooms, broccoli, lentils, grapefruits, peanuts, spinach, chard, and celery are all examples of this. Broccoli, lentils, and grapefruit have naturally occurring pesticides, which, if you extracted and ate in their concentrated forms in high doses, can cause mutations. Mushrooms contain carcinogens. Peanuts can harbor traces of aflatoxin, cancer-causing substances. Spinach and chard contain an acid that can diminish calcium absorption. And celery has toxins that can damage the immune system.[327] But these are all healthy foods. And the sums of all their parts offer protection from the potential dangers of one or two individual components. It's when we start tinkering with their chemistry that we see "dangers." So it isn't surprising to see breast cancer cells in mice who are dosed with a thousand milligrams of soy isoflavones.

Another common accusation is that soy has a negative impact on thyroid function. However, only one adult human study conducted in Japan over fifteen years ago has concluded that. (And better-designed and more recent studies done in the United States did not support those findings.)[328] Every day for three months straight, seventeen people were fed thirty grams of pickled, roasted soybeans. Half of these participants experienced either an enlargement of the thyroid *or* a hypothyroidism symptom, like fatigue or constipation.[329] Do eight or nine people (some experiencing only fatigue or constipation) prove that soy has a negative effect on thyroid function?

The Myths and Lies About Protein

So a lot of the negative hype around soy is bullshit. Does that mean soy is the wonder bean and will cure baldness, burn fat, and make your wang-doodle bigger? We have no idea. And we're not interested in delving deeper into any research that makes these claims. In our humble opinions based on research we trust, moderate consumption of soy products is safe. Do we eat ten servings a day? No. Do we take soy supplements? No. Do we add soy powders to our smoothies? No. Do we use soy as a wonder food or drug? No. But do we eat soy products? Yep.

We're not medical researchers or epidemiologists, so we'll understand if our humble opinions don't mean shit to you. According to health expert Dr. Andrew Weil, "There is still much to be learned about soy, but the majority of research so far has shown that it's a safe and nutritious food when eaten in reasonable amounts—about one or two daily servings."[335] And even though countless other doctors, medical researchers, and epidemiologists also feel moderate consumption of soy products is safe, their opinions may not mean shit to you, either. Good! You're questioning authority and taking matters into your own hands! We encourage you to think for yourself and make your own decisions. (Or let your nag-ass wife decide for you.) If you're still not sure about soy, do your own research and decide for yourself, especially if you or your family members have thyroid problems or breast cancer. Knowledge is *self*-power. Kowtowing to your doctor without doing your own homework is just plain lazy. But be prepared to dig deep for the truth. Some pro-soy medical studies are paid for by the soy industry. Some anti-soy medical studies are paid for by the dairy and meat industries.

If you decide to eat soy products, know that these foods may not taste exactly like the real thing. But once you get rid of your meat addiction, you'll be satisfied with the substitutes. You just need to spend a few weeks (and dollars) experimenting until you find the ones you like. Veggie burgers exist by the dozen. Health Is Wealth makes fake buffalo wings that taste so good, your pubes will fall out. Gardenburger's flame-grilled chik'n is so amazing, you might have to kill yourself. Lightlife and Tofurky have kick-ass lines of "cold cuts" and incredible "bacon." And Gardein has it all! Seek and ye shall find. You don't have to look far: We list these meatless wonders in Chapter 12.

Remember to use common sense, too. In general, the more processed a food is, the less wholesome it is for you. (Like eating an apple and a handful of nuts is healthier than eating an energy bar that has apple and nuts in it.) So whole soybeans, edamame, tofu, tempeh, and miso are more nutritious than other more highly processed soy foods. But if faced with eating chicken or soy chicken, meat or soy meat, cheese or soy cheese, we'd definitely choose the soy every time. (FYI: Many people find soy products to be excellent transitional foods for getting off meat and dairy products. Then, after a few months or even a year, they discontinue eating soy.) But also remember that it doesn't have to be either/or. You can abstain from eating animal products *and* soy and still be healthy. So long as you are eating a balance of fruits, veggies, whole grains, legumes, nuts, and seeds every day, and following doctors' orders for supplementing, you will thrive.

An integral part of any healthy, balanced diet is fat. Don't cringe. Fat doesn't always mean fattening. Essential fatty acids provide us with energy and offer protection from heart disease, stroke, and high blood pressure. They also combat allergies, arthritis, and skin problems.[336] Our brilliant bodies make all the essential fatty acids we need, except for two: linoleic and linolenic acids, also known as omega-3 and omega-6.[337] These *good fats* are found in nuts, seeds (and their "butters"), olives, avocados, and olive oil, sesame oil, flaxseed oil, canola oil, and hempseed oil. So quit listening to all the stupid pansies who boycott nuts, oils, and avocados because they think they're fattening. Even though they're high in fat, they will not make you fat (unless you overdose on them). Unsaturated fats such as these are good for your body, and when eaten as part of a well-balanced vegan diet, they don't make you fat! It's the saturated fats found in meat, dairy, and hydrogenated oils that make you fat. Think about the source of the oils or fats and use your head. Do you think an avocado, which is a fruit, is going to turn you into a lardass? Common sense, dude.

Speaking of common sense, now that you're totally onboard with the whole veg thing, we need to point something out to you: People are really fucking stupid when it comes to vegetarianism; they just can't wrap their minds around it. Everyone has a preconceived notion about it and it's really hard for them to step outside what they think they know. You will inevitably come up against one, if not all of, the following ridiculous statements:

* *"I knew a vegetarian once—he was fat; he ate a ton of junk food all the time."*

Um, I know about a million meat-eaters who are fat and eat a ton of junk food all the time.

The Myths and Lies About Protein

* *"I've seen plenty of pale, skinny, unhealthy-looking vegetarians."*

Hmm…there is no shortage of pale, skinny, unhealthy-looking meat-eaters.

* *"I could never give up eating meat."*

Um, no one is asking you to, narcissist, I'm just telling you that I don't eat it.

* *"Oh, I wouldn't go vegetarian; vegetarians don't get enough protein."*

Actually, they get plenty. But it's always fascinating how people express concern about protein deficiency, as opposed to real issues, like heart disease, diabetes, and cancers—our nation's top killers, all of which meat-eaters are more likely to encounter.

Ah, people. They can be idiots. Forgive them. They know not how dumb they are.

Chapter 8

No Girls Allowed

Hypertension and Heart Disease— Man's Worst Enemy

We pity you men, we do. We know that we women are impossible to please; we can nag like nobody's business; and no matter how much times change or how much the gender equality gap closes, men still feel the weight of the world on their shoulders. You're "selfish," "you don't make enough money," "you work too much," "you don't spend enough time with the kids," "you aren't romantic enough," "you care more about golf than me," blah, blah, blah, blah, blah, blah, blah. It's challenging not to let life (and your wife) get to you. But you really need to figure out how to be more Zen—stress is a definite factor in causing high blood pressure.[338] There are other contributors, too, like alcohol, poor nutrition, poor fitness, and Type A personality traits.[339] Just so we're all on the same page, here's how it works: "Doctors measure blood pressure using two numbers, such as 120/80. The first number shows the surge of pressure in the arteries with every beat, and the second number shows the pressure between beats."[340] If either one of those numbers is too high, it's bad news bears.[341] High blood pressure is known as "the silent killer" because approximately 40 percent of Americans who have it go undiagnosed.[342] Some early warning signs may include fainting, dizziness, blurry vision, ringing in the ears, nosebleeds, flushing of the face, headaches (especially in the morning), and tension when there is no cause.[343] If you do suffer from high blood pressure, the good news is that 85 percent of all cases can be reversed, just through changes in diet and lifestyle.[344] (For starters, lay off the salt and high-sodium foods. FYI: canned food is notorious for being high in sodium.)[345] If you don't get a handle on it, high blood pressure will lead to heart disease.[346]

Heart disease is the deadliest killer in the United States, nabbing one out of three Americans.[347] And while it's killing both sexes, annually, thousands more men die of heart disease than women, and at a younger age.[348] One of the reasons heart disease is so pervasive is that two-thirds of Americans are overweight.[349] Smoking and drinking are also contributors, of course.[350] Yes, heart disease can also be hereditary, but only about 5 percent of the population has a true genetic disposition.[351] So quit blaming bad genes.

Instead, blame your high cholesterol, which is of your own doing. Cholesterol, a waxy substance, is an essential component of the membrane that coats all our cells.[352] It's also the basic ingredient of our sex hormones.[353] So you get why we need it, and thankfully, our bodies produce it. What we don't need is to consume foods that have cholesterol in them, because they tend to raise our bad cholesterol. And it just so happens that the foods that have cholesterol in them are animal-based foods (meat, chicken, fish, eggs, dairy).[354] So if you thought "lean cuts" were low in cholesterol, think again—the cholesterol is mainly in the lean portion.[355] And if you thought chicken was "health food," think again—chicken has as much cholesterol as beef.[356] Whether it's beef or chicken, four ounces means 100 milligrams of cholesterol![357] When you have "high cholesterol," the waxy substance can build up on the walls of the arteries. Eventually, the arteries get clogged. Think about your body for a moment. Think about how your arteries are blood vessels, responsible for supplying oxygen and nutrients to your entire body. Now imagine your arteries being clogged up so that your healthy, nutrient-rich, oxygenated blood cannot freely flow throughout your body. Imagine all the toxic gunk and junk that gets formed and that starts circulating through your body. Are you able to see how little by little, slowly but surely, you're doing an incredible amount of damage to yourself? When the sludge builds up to the point that it blocks a blood vessel to the heart, it's a heart attack, and when it blocks a blood vessel to the brain, it's a stroke. You're sabotaging your whole body, your overall health and vitality, and your life. P. S. High cholesterol also means a higher likelihood of impotence,[358] so you're also jeopardizing your Johnson!

Don't Mess with Diabetes

Not only are obesity and heart disease on the rise, but so is diabetes, affecting 1 out of 13 Americans (with that ratio continuing to increase).[359] According to Dr. Campbell, "Both diabetes and obesity are merely symptoms of poor health in general. They rarely exist in isolation of other diseases and often forecast deeper, more serious health problems, such as heart disease, cancer, and stroke. Two of the most frightening statistics show that diabetes among people in their thirties has increased 70 percent in less than ten years and the percentage of obese people has nearly doubled in the past thirty years."[360] Both are diet related. You do not want to mess with diabetes. It can cause stroke, heart disease, kidney disease, gum disease (which can lead to tooth loss), damage to the nervous system, blindness, and amputation.[361] Maybe that burger or chicken sandwich tastes good, but good enough to give up your sight or your leg? If you already have diabetes, don't despair. One of the most prominent scientists in the field of diet and diabetes is Dr. James Anderson. One of his studies included fifty people with diabetes—twenty-five who were Type 1 and twenty-five who were Type 2. (Type 1s cannot produce adequate insulin to manage the transport and distribution of glucose, Type 2s can produce insulin, but their insulin doesn't work properly.)[362] All of the people in the study were using insulin and none were overweight. After three weeks of Dr. Anderson's experimental "veggie" diet (mostly whole plant foods and the equivalent of only a cold cut or two a day), the results were staggering. Not only did their cholesterol levels drop 30 percent, the Type 1s were also able to reduce their insulin intake by an average of 40 percent![363] The Type 2s had even better results: twenty-four out of the twenty-five were able to stop taking insulin in a matter of weeks![364] All because they changed their diets!

Smoking, drinking, being sedentary, and eating a shitty diet of meat, dairy, and processed foods will eventually catch up to you. It's not like breaking your arm, where you feel the effects right away. It's cumulative, and you may not know how much damage you're doing until you get some scary news from your doctor. So don't wait to get diagnosed with a deadly disease.

Size Matters

The prostate, a small organ about the size of a walnut, is responsible for producing some of your seminal fluid. And in this instance, bigger is *not* better—an enlarged prostate could mean trouble. The last thing you want to hear is that you have prostate cancer, especially when you could've easily prevented it—diet plays a key role in the disease.[365] A 2001 Harvard review of multiple studies clearly states that dairy "is one of the most consistent dietary predictors for prostate cancer."[366] Men who consume high amounts of dairy increase their risk for prostate cancer by a whopping 70 percent![367] Most dairy products are high in fat, which affects the sex hormones that can cause cancer.[368] But the fat-free bullshit is no better. According to an article in *Alternative Medicine Reviews*, worldwide, prostate cancer is more closely linked to nonfat dairy products than any other food.[369] A different review of twenty-three studies revealed, "animal protein, meats, dairy products and eggs have frequently been associated with a higher risk of prostate cancer . . ."[370] Here's one way it happens: We all have this hormone in our bodies, Insulin-like Growth Factor 1 (IGF-1). Under normal conditions, IGF-1 keeps our cells reproducing at a healthy rate and helps rid our bodies of old cells. It's this healthy growing of new cells and discarding of old cells that keep us cancer-free. But when we eat meat and dairy, our IGF-1 level increases, disturbing the balance of new cell growth and old cell removal, leading to . . .[371] ca-ca-ca-cancer. Not only is IGF-1 naturally present in our bodies, but it's also present in dairy products.[372] No wonder men who consume dairy regularly have increased levels of IGF-1 in their bodies.[373] A recent study comparing men's IGF-1 levels showed those who tested highest to be at *four times* the risk for prostate cancer than those who tested lowest.[374] There are other studies linking the high amount of calcium in dairy with having a negative impact on the body's vitamin D situation (which is thought to provide protection against prostate cancer).[375]

Another possible cause of prostate cancer is the high amount of environmental toxins (pesticides, industrial pollutants, etc.) present in dairy[376] and meat.[377] Or, it could be the cooking of these foods. All foods that are broiled or fried contain mutagens, chemicals that can do cellular damage.[378] But animal foods have far more mutagens than similarly cooked plant foods.[379]

Dr. William Castelli, director of the Framingham Health Study (the longest-running study of diet and heart disease in the world), said, "Vegetarians have the best diet; they have the lowest rates of coronary heart disease of any group in the country."[380] Of his groundbreaking work/book, *The China Study,* the most comprehensive study of diet and disease in medical history, Dr. Colin Campbell said, "People who ate the most animal-based foods got the most chronic disease. Even relatively small intakes of animal-based foods were associated with adverse effects. People who ate the most plant-based foods were the healthiest and tended to avoid chronic disease."[381]

So there you have it. Abstaining from animal foods will do you a world of good—for prevention of high blood pressure, heart disease, obesity, diabetes, and cancer. But you've got to eat plant foods, too— for prevention of high blood pressure, heart disease, obesity, diabetes, and cancer. Fruits, vegetables, whole grains, nuts, seeds, and legumes can dramatically reduce risk of heart disease;[382] protect against cancer, stop cancer, and reverse cancer;[383] and neutralize the free radicals.[384]

Plant foods are like friggin' magic. Seriously. Men with *low* levels of beta-carotene have a 45 percent increased risk for prostate cancer. So eating apricots, carrots, sweet potatoes, and yams can reduce risk.[385] Men who eat lycopene-rich foods (tomatoes are the best source) have a 45 percent reduced risk for getting prostate cancer![386] (Don't try to cheat the system by taking some lycopene supplement. Studies aren't conclusive if supplements are as beneficial as getting lycopene from food sources.[387] In our opinion, you can't trick Mother Nature.) Eating cruciferous veggies like broccoli, Brussels sprouts, cauliflower, and kale reduces risk by 41 percent![388] No wonder vegetarian men have low rates of prostate cancer![389] The lucky fellas who were raised vegetarian have the lowest risk of all.[390]

Strap on a Pair

Yes, women want men to be sensitive and in touch with their feminine sides. But we still want you to be friggin' men, so you better be sure you're producing the right amount of testosterone. Not only is testosterone responsible for your muscles, manly voice, and facial and body hair, but it's also key for your sex drive, sperm production, and sexual function.[391] Some possible symptoms of low testosterone levels can include fatigue, depression, irritability (hey, bitch), reduced strength, reduced muscle mass, low sex drive, and erectile dysfunction.[392] If you lost your woody during sex last week, don't go jumping off a bridge. Shit happens, and it doesn't necessarily mean you have low testosterone. But if you think your testes may be in troubs, there a few easy, safe, natural ways to get your nads back on track. For starters, lose some weight, bub. Researchers found that going from non-obese to obese can cause a testosterone-reduction equal to *ten years* of aging.[393] Oy vey. Significant extra poundage not only causes a decrease in testosterone, but it can also cause an increase in estrogen.[394] (Hey, man-boobs.) But don't freak out and try to lose fifty pounds overnight. If you start exercising too much and eating too little, your body will think it's starving and will stop producing testosterone.[395] Talk about counterproductive. Definitely exercise, though. Cardio, which is good for weight loss and your heart, can also help reduce stress. And stress can cause cortisol (stress hormone) levels to surge, hampering your testosterone production.[396] So move it, mister! And while you're at it, hit the racks. Regular weight lifting will not only give you manly muscles, but it's also been shown to dramatically increase testosterone levels.[397] Some studies have suggested that doing multi-joint exercises that work large muscle groups (squats, dead-lifts, bench presses, etc.) are better testosterone boosters than single-joint, small muscle exercises.[398] Regardless of what you do, don't overdo it! Research has shown that overtraining can reduce testosterone.[399] (Kinda makes you wonder about all those freaky muscle-heads . . . little pee-pees?) Be sure to eat a well-balanced diet, too. A Penn State study revealed that a high-protein/low-carb diet can have a negative impact on testosterone levels.[400] (Surprise, surprise.) So, of course, load up on fruits, veggies, whole grains, and legumes, and make sure you're also getting enough healthy fats from nuts, seeds, and avocados. According to research, men who eat healthy, monounsaturated fats have hearty levels of testosterone.[401] And do your best to eat organic. Pesticides have been linked to a decline in testosterone.[402] One interesting study found that a group of organic farmers had sperm counts *twice as high* as men in a control group of blue-collar workers, suggesting organic foods may be good for your boys.[403]

Locker Room Talk

So clearly, you want to make sure you do what you need to do to keep your hormones in check. That way, you'll keep your man-glue in check. Men who booze excessively or do drugs (yes, pot is a drug) can have compromised sperm count and quality.[404] Men who let their junk get too heated too often are also at risk. Hot baths and spa-use shouldn't be excessive, and you really shouldn't work with your laptop on your lap.[405] All can affect your jis, as can wearing underwear that's too tight.[406] So swap out your little girl bikini panties for some boxers or others loose-fitting numbers. FYI: Not only does smoking affect your sperm,[407] but it also affects your virility. Almost two-thirds of impotent men smoke.[408] And get this: Studies have shown that the number of ciggies smoked is directly proportional to the blood flow decrease in the cockadoodledo.[409] Crazy! (But not really—it makes perfect sense.) So quit smoking, stupid! It's messing with your stick! If you do discover that you have spastic sperm even after quitting smoking, eating well, exercising, and avoiding having your balls scorched, try acupuncture. It's been shown to have a positive impact on sperm count, shape, and movement.[410]

Tangy Taste Test?

By the way, since we're already talking about all your private business, it just has to be said: You are what you eat. Meaning, your diet and lifestyle affect the smell and taste of your man juice. Think about it. Unhealthy people who smoke and eat crap and drink coffee tend to have smelly body odor, shitty breath, and foul-stinking piss. Why would their *other* secretions be any different? (BTW: Vegans typically have better breath than meat-eaters. The digestion of animal protein creates a bacterial environment, which is not so fresh-smelling.)[411] Only about one percent of what you unload is sperm, which you wouldn't really expect to have a certain smell. But as for the other 99 percent, what do you think would make it smell good? Beer? Coffee? Processed, chemical, fake foods? The rotting, decomposing, putrefying carcass of a slaughtered animal? Nasty-ass curdled milk or cheese? Grooooooooooss! If you don't believe that diet affects your spooge, play our thirty-day goo game. Today, having eaten the way you normally do, do the deed, and then smell your stuff. Funky gunk, right? For the next thirty days, eat a pure, healthy diet like we prescribe in this book. At the end of the month, whack and sniff. Your love nectar's scent will be so much better, you'll likely be tempted to taste it!

Move It!

Exercise can dramatically reduce risk of high blood pressure,[412] heart disease,[413] prostate cancer,[414] obesity, stroke, diabetes, memory loss, colon cancer, fractures, depression, and erectile dysfunction.[415] And you don't have to become an Ironman to reap the benefits. One study of more than 15,000 men found that "the risk of death is cut in half with an exercise capacity that can easily be achieved by a brisk walk of about 30 minutes per session five to six days per week."[416]

Of course you should consult your doctor before beginning any exercise regimen, but especially if you're about to turn into one of those crazy, bodybuilding freaks. The human body, when treated well, can function like a perfect machine. So first and foremost, be honest with yourself about what kind of machine you are. Some men are designed to be diesel mo'fos; others, to run like the wind; and others, to just be fit and healthy. While we clearly live in a society that is obsessed with looks, do your best to aim for *fitness* goals, and not *appearance* goals. That way, you will be working smart, doing good for your body, and enjoying the process. And of course, it is likely your body will look better, too. But all of us (even men) have skewed perceptions of how we look. So don't allow your desire to look a certain way drive your efforts. Aim to get strong and healthy and fit from the inside out. Yes, our culture idolizes athletes, but these sports gods really aren't all that enviable. Their bodies take tremendous abuse, and they suffer lifetimes of chronic pain and problems as a result. Training at such high levels is a huge stressor and can often be very physically damaging.

So now that you're ready to exercise at a healthy level, here's what you need to know:

Drink a shitload of water. Yeah, yeah, yeah, everyone knows that water is clutch, but do you really do a good job of staying hydrated? It's bad when you don't drink enough water in real life, but it's even worse when you don't drink enough during exercise. Not only is it vital for

No Girls Allowed

proper organ function, but it's also imperative for cardiovascular health, body temperature maintenance, muscle function,[417] and for staving off muscle cramps, fatigue, dizziness, heat stroke, and heat exhaustion.[418] Start hydrating two to three hours before exercise, with about 15–20 ounces of water; then, fifteen minutes before exercise, have about 8 ounces more.[419] (But don't chug it all at once— you'll get bloated.) And of course, make sure to continue drinking while you're exercising. You don't have to take big swigs in the middle of your work-out and give yourself a stomach cramp, but you want to be consciously hydrating. Approximately 8 ounces every fifteen minutes during exercise should do the trick.[420] But because each person's weight, exercise level, and sweat output are different, there's no perfect water prescription that applies to everyone. However, there are two good ways to gauge your own water needs. First off, take a look at your piss. If there's a lot of it, it's light in color, and it's diluted-looking, good job. If it's a scant amount, dark in color, and it looks concentrated, you're not drinking enough.[421] Second, weigh yourself just before and after exercising. Immediate weight loss is likely water weight, so you need to be drinking more.[422] For every pound lost, try to replenish with 20–24 ounces of water.[423]

But be careful not to drown yourself in an effort to stay hydrated. There's a condition called hyponatremia, also known as *water intoxication*. When the body loses too much sodium, drinking plain water can even further dilute sodium levels.[424] It's in these cases of extreme, high intensity exercise and perspiration that sports drinks may come in handy. But just so you know, a lot of them are crap. If you eat a well-balanced diet; stay hydrated before, during and after workouts; and don't exercise for more than sixty minutes at a high intensity, you should be fine without a sports drink.[425] However, if you're working out like a fiend and you do need to replenish electrolytes, choose a sports drink that doesn't have artificial flavors, artificial colors, artificial sweeteners, or caffeine. None of those serve your health.

Eating for Action

At this point in the book, you should know that a vegan diet is the healthiest way to go. And that if you're just a regular guy who wants to eat well, be healthy, go the gym, and look good, you just need to eat a well-balanced vegan diet and all your butch dreams can come true. You should also know that veganism allows you to be an ass-kicking warrior, whatever your sport of choice. Veganism does not translate to men in Birkenstocks wearing patchouli, weighing ten pounds, and talking about their feelings. (Of course we do have a few of those, much to the chagrin of all the vegan women.) Go back and read the list of all the veggie jocks we mentioned earlier—athletes at the top of their games who are tough-ass sons of bitches. Those guys are beasts, and you can be, too. There are a few good books on the subject of veggie athleticism and training, so go get one for a more detailed overview.

But here's a tiny, little peek into the lives of veggie athletes: For starters, they frickin' love carbs. Years of solid research have shown the benefits of plant-based, high-carb diets for athletic performance. Studies consistently show that at about the same time that glycogen stores get low, fatigue sets in.[426] Because high-carb diets maximize liver and glycogen stores, endurance and energy levels are optimized,[427] which means decreased risk of muscle- and whole-body fatigue; increased stamina; and increased energy reserves for that final sprint, tackle, pin, hit, basket, or goal.[428] Complex carbs also help prevent dehydration, since they absorb water.[429] Just a reminder, complex carbs are fruits, veggies, whole grains, legumes, nuts, and seeds. Admittedly, sometimes the "bulkiness" of complex carbs right before a race can cause gas, bloating, and pooping at inopportune times.[430] So if you're a marathoner or other serious competitor, you'll have to experiment with your diet and timing. But know that according to the American Dietetic Association, the Canadian Dietetic Association, and Dieticians of Canada, for physical fitness and athletic performance, approximately 60–70 percent of your calories should come from carbs.[431]

But that doesn't mean you should forsake fat. Fat is important for everyday civilians and athletes. Yes, fat can make you fat if you just eat tons of fat and sit around being fat. But fat is a major energy resource (especially for distance events); the source of essential fatty acids (EFAs); and a carrier of vitamins, minerals, and phytochemcials.[432] While there's no substitute for carbs, the body can store far more energy as fat than as glycogen—both within muscle cells and around the body's cells.[433] The flab stored within your muscles is readily available for aerobic activity.[434] We constantly need to replenish our carb stores, but our fat stores are always there for the using. And the best sources for healthy, unsaturated fats are avocados, olives, raw nuts, raw seeds, raw nut butters, flax seed oil, hemp seed oil, and extra-virgin olive oil—all organic, of course. (If you have heart disease or it runs in your family, you may need to skip the oils altogether; check with your cardiologist. Actually, since he or she literally may not know shit about diet, read Dr. Caldwell Esselstyn's book *Preventing and Reversing Heart Disease* first, then talk to your doctor. Dr. Esselstyn's work is revolutionary, mind-blowing, and life altering.)

Before we talk about protein, we want to remind you, again, that it's not the end-all, be-all—so keep it in your pants. Yes, people who are active may need more protein than couch potatoes. Yes, protein is an integral energy source and it's imperative for muscle tissue growth, maintenance, and repair.[435] Yes, it can be damaging to your muscles if you don't get adequate protein.[436] That said, the general recommendation for protein intake for vegan athletes is about 12–15 percent.[437] Of course, that percentage can go up or down, considering caloric intake, energy output, and fitness activities and goals.[438] Now just so we're clear, when we say the recommended amount for "athletes," we mean those who are training intensely for eight to forty hours a week, especially if you're starting a new regimen or if it's the beginning of the season.[439] These recommended amounts are not for fitness enthusiasts or guys who are just recreationally active. Again, this is a general book about health and diet, so if you want to get all cuckoo for calories, fat, and protein and start training for an Ironman, there are much better books to help guide you on that journey. But know that it is possible to get too much protein (even if you're a vegan) if you start supplementing with all those protein powders.[440] Remember, high intensity activities can take a lot out of you, whether you're a meat-eater or vegan. So if you need astronomical amounts of protein just to survive those feats, perhaps you should reconsider. Plus, drinking some gritty-ass shake is hardly as fun as pigging out. Some high protein foods include nuts, beans, quinoa (a grain), seitan (a "meat" made from wheat), tofu, veggie burgers, and tempeh (fermented soy).[441]

It's a funny thing, this eating for fitness. All the plant foods we keep mentioning not only have the good fat, protein, and carbs you need, but they're also good sources for vitamins and minerals. As an athlete, you may need to supplement (talk to your doctor), but don't get all performance-focused on us. These aren't for performance-enhancing purposes, they're for your health and protection. Studies have suggested that athletes may require increased vitamin C, which is especially important for connective tissue.[442] The B vitamins help metabolize energy, process amino acids, and synthesize new cells.[443] For a vegan, B-12 is always an important one to stay on top of. And as a general precaution, it's good to investigate your vitamin D situation and make sure you're up to snuff. Vegan or not, low iron is the most common deficiency issue for athletes,[444] so be sure you're getting enough. (Eating iron-rich foods with vitamin C-rich foods helps with absorption.) Because too much iron can be damaging, have your levels checked before deciding whether to pop a pill.[445] Calcium levels can be compromised in some athletes due to poor dietary intake and intense training—calcium gets used during muscle contractions.[446] Vegan athletes usually do okay because they consume calcium-rich foods and fortified soy- and rice milks; however, you may need to up your intake depending on your workout.[447] You certainly don't want to be sidelined by fractures, muscle problems, or nerve issues.[448] Zinc is important for tissue repair, but can be depleted through urine and sweat.[449] But vegans who eat legumes, nuts, seeds, and whole grains on a daily basis should be fine.[450]

So whether you want to get a little buff, crazy jacked-up, or just plain healthy, eating a well-balanced vegan diet of whole plant foods makes it all possible. You'll see and feel the difference when you try it for yourself.

After that, if you still don't get it, we give up. Just go be a dumb jock somewhere.

Chapter 9

Dumping

Pinch a loaf. Lay a cable. Drop a deuce. Let's face it; there is no greater pleasure than taking a big, steamy dump. But shitting isn't just for kicks. It is a vital tool for weight loss and optimal health. Basic math. How much are you putting in your mouth, and how much is coming out your ass? Now that you've learned the right foods to eat and which ones to avoid, you should be a dynamo in the bathroom. But if your hiney is expelling only little rabbit turds, something's gotta give.

Earlier, we mentioned that drinking lots of water helps rid your body of waste. We can't emphasize the importance of this enough. Drink, drink, drink. But if you want to take tyrannosaurus-sized dumps, it's also imperative to eat foods rich in fiber, like whole-grain cereals and breads, brown rice, corn, barley, rye, buckwheat, millet, oats, fruits, vegetables (especially root vegetables, like carrots), beans, and seeds. Avoid foods that have little or no fiber, like meat, eggs, cheese, milk, and processed, refined foods. These can clog up your ass.

Fiber isn't just for shits and giggles, either. It offers protection from appendicitis, heart disease, high blood pressure, high cholesterol, diabetes, gallstones, irritable bowel syndrome, and colitis.[451] Fibrous foods also help normalize our blood-sugar levels, sate food cravings, and make us feel fuller so that we don't overeat.[452] Fiber even fights colon, colorectal, and prostate cancer: If we don't make ca-ca quickly enough, our putrefying food stays in our bodies, increasing the likelihood of the production of carcinogenic substances. So eat your fiber, and crap like a champ.[453] Another way to get your bowels brewing is to pay special attention to the order in which you are eating foods. For example, foods that digest quickly and easily should be eaten by themselves and early in the day. Fruit for breakfast. Salad and/or vegetables for lunch. These foods will pass through your body at lightning speeds. Dinner should be your "heaviest" meal. Follow these simple rules, and you'll be depositing six-inchers in no time. If you're already a quality dumper, feel free to disregard.

But, if you still need an extra kick in the ass, up your bean intake.

Beware: You might have a mudslide in your pants if you're not careful. If you're not accustomed to beans, ease in slowly so your body can get used to digesting them. Expect some noise, for sure. And hey, maybe even stay close to a toilet to play it safe.

If your log-laying still needs work, do not take laxatives. Yes, they make you poop, but they don't solve the underlying problem of why you're not pooping in the first place. Most laxatives are gastrointestinal irritants—even the natural ones.[454] Stop looking for a quick fix. Just continue to drink a lot of water, exercise, and eat right, shitheads.

Chapter 10

Have No Faith:
The Government Doesn't
Give a Shit
About Your Health

The USDA: It's Not What You Think

President Abraham Lincoln founded the U.S. Department of Agriculture in 1862—when the majority of people were farmers and needed to exchange information about seeds and crops. In other words, the USDA was created to help farmers.

Now, among other things, the USDA is responsible for "the safety of meat, poultry, and egg products."[455]

Hmm. That's weird. 'Cause many high-ranking staff members at the USDA were employed by, or are otherwise affiliated with, the meat and dairy industries.[457] And if the group responsible for "the safety of meat, poultry, and egg products" is run by people from the same industries they're supposed to be protecting us from . . . well, that would be a conflict of interest. *And it is.* An enormous, ridiculous, outrageous, catastrophic conflict of interest.

One former USDA secretary was forced to resign amid charges of accepting illegal corporate gifts from seven different companies. He was indicted on thirty-nine felony counts, including tampering with a witness, accepting illegal gratuities, making false statements, and violating the Meat Inspection Act of 1907. (Tyson Foods, one of the companies that admitted to giving the secretary corporate favors, was required to pay $4 million in fines and endure four years' probation. A mere slap on the wrist, when the USDA could've barred Tyson from selling food to military bases and schools. That would've really stung, considering Tyson sold more than $10 million worth of food to the Defense Department alone in 1996.[458] But friends don't treat each other that way.)

President George W. Bush's Agriculture secretary from January 2001 until January 2005, Ann Veneman, not only had ties with the company responsible for producing the controversial bovine growth hormone, she was also linked to a major meatpacking corporation.[459] It doesn't stop there. She employed a spokeswoman who is the former public relations director for the National Cattlemen's Beef Association, a chief of staff who used to be its head lobbyist, a former president of the National Pork Producers Council, and former executives from the meatpacking industry, just to name a few.[460]

Safety Last

With that in mind, it's no wonder Veneman vetoed a program that would test all U.S. cattle for mad cow disease. In fact, out of the 35 million cattle slaughtered in 2003, the USDA tested only 20,000 for mad cow disease. (Japan tests *all* of its cattle killed for human consumption.)[461] Of course it wouldn't be in a rancher's best interest to test all of his cattle. If they were inflicted with mad cow disease, he couldn't sell their meat, and he'd lose money. Heaven forbid the USDA risk a rancher's profits.

So, to appear somewhat concerned about the prevention of mad cow disease, the USDA often refers to an FDA ban, which prohibits the feeding of ground-up cattle meat to live cattle. Big whoop.

Banning cannibalism is a no-brainer. But why even bother banning cannibalism when they still allow the feeding of *cattle blood* to young calves? Stanley Prusiner, a Nobel Prize winner for his work on mad cow disease, refers to this practice as "a really stupid idea."[462] Think about it: A cow dies from mad cow disease, but no one knows, because it wasn't one of the .05714 percent tested. Cattle ranchers are now forbidden to grind up this dead cow and feed it to other cows. But they can give its blood to calves as part of their feed. How fucking stupid, disgusting, and dangerous is that?

The USDA also likes referring to another "safety" program in place called the National Animal Identification System (NAIS). The NAIS is a system for identifying an animal's origin so that if its meat is found to be contaminated, it can be traced back to a specific farm. (Forget testing as a preventive measure. Implement a system for *after* someone eats contaminated meat and we need a recall.) Participation in this program is *voluntary*.[463] Wow, the USDA sure has tough rules governing the safety of our country's meat.

The USDA's website describing the NAIS actually has a section on "confidentiality." It reads, "The NAIS will contain only information necessary for animal health officials to be able to track suspect animals and identify any other animals that may have been exposed to a disease. . . . To help assure participants that the information will be used only for animal health purposes, the information must be confidential. USDA and its state partners will work to protect data confidentiality."[464] What the fuck? The USDA will protect the data confidentiality of farms that are supplying the public with contaminated meat? Why don't they just give all the ranchers blowjobs, too?

Many savvy consumers are catching on, and they know they cannot trust the USDA. According to the Organic Consumers Association, "Lester Friedlander, a former USDA veterinarian, says he was told by USDA officials as far back as 1991 that if his testing ever found evidence of mad cow disease, he was to tell no one. He and other scientists say they know of cases where cows tested positive for the disease in laboratories but were ruled negative by the USDA."[465] Trust no one!

Illegal hormones, which are suspected of increasing the growth of cancer cells in the humans who eat them, are regularly pumped into veal calves. The USDA has not only been accused of overlooking these practices but also of falsifying lab results, altering records, and pressuring staff to lie about events.[466] Even the selfish assholes who eat veal don't deserve that.

Business First

None of us has deserved to be deceived all these years by the pre-
posterous USDA Dietary Guidelines and Food Pyramid, either. In
1998, the Physicians Committee for Responsible Medicine (PCRM)
sued the USDA and the Department of Health and Human Services.
PCRM claimed that federal laws were violated when the USDA
selected six out of eleven people with financial ties to various food
industries to serve on the Dietary Guidelines Advisory Committee.
The committee members' affiliations included the American Meat
Institute, National Livestock and Beef Board, the American Egg
Board, the National Dairy Promotion and Research Program, the
National Dairy Council, Dannon Company (yogurt), Mead Johnson
Nutritionals (milk-based infant formulas), Nestlé (milk-based formu-
las, ice cream, condensed milk), and Slim-Fast (milk-based diet
products).[467] How dare they?

PCRM also charged that the Dietary Guidelines—which recommended dairy products—were racially biased because most
nonwhites are lactose intolerant.[468] According to Johnson & Johnson,
lactose intolerance affects "over 50 percent of the Hispanic American
population, 75 percent of Native Americans, 80 percent of African

Have No Faith

Americans, and 90 percent of Asian Americans."[469] Why does Johnson & Johnson care about the millions of minorities suffering from lactose intolerance? Because they can target these individuals for buying Lactaid, a product they hawk for aiding in dairy digestion. Even though you are lactose *intolerant* and your body thoroughly rejects dairy products, eat them anyway. Just buy and take our drug so you don't feel sick afterward. Ugh, that just makes us sick with rage.

Got $50 billion? The milk industry does, so they've got the USDA in their back pocket.[470] The California Milk Processor Board (CMPB) was established in 1993 to increase milk sales in California. They were responsible for the campaigns that targeted children: "Got milk?" and "Milk. It does a body good." The CMPB is funded by all California milk processors but administered by the California Department of Food and Agriculture. The National Fluid Milk Processor Promotion Board (Fluid Board) conceived of the "Milk Mustache" campaign, which targets young adults. The USDA's Agriculture Monitoring Service administers the Fluid Board.[471] Meaning, in essence, the California Department of Agriculture and the USDA are managing advertising campaigns for the milk industry. Under the guise of advancing health, they managed to dupe President Bill Clinton while he was in office into posing for their ads. They also had the audacity to feature the Secretary of Health and Human Services, Donna Shalala, sporting that stupid "milk mustache."[472] The Secretary of Health and Human Services using her status and title to promote a commercial product! Would she appear in ads for Pepsi or Nike? Say it out loud: conflict of interest. They've even got the U.S. Surgeon General in on the act. In the first-ever report on "the state of the nation's bones," the Surgeon General warned of an impending "osteoporosis crisis" expected by the year 2020. To ward off this potential disaster, the report recommended three glasses of milk a day. Guess who issued the report? The Department of Health and Human Services.[473] Ughck. In 2007, the "Body By Milk" campaign suggested that three servings of dairy per day would help people lose weight. They even enlisted NY Yankee, Alex Rodriguez, to help out. But according to the Federal Trade Commission, scientific research did not support the dairy industry's claim, and thankfully, the campaign was ended.[474] Trust no one.

The horrors committed by the USDA could fill an entire book. But we shouldn't be surprised. Although they don't list it as part of their primary mission statement, the USDA admits to being "committed to helping America's farmers and ranchers."[475] The same USDA responsible for "the safety" of meat, poultry, dairy, and eggs also promotes the sale of them. In fact, they even go so far as to purchase the products themselves, using our tax dollars. In 2005, the government spent $385 million on beef and cheese (yet only about $50 million for fresh fruits and vegetables).[476] Farmers growing fruits and veggies received less than 1 percent of direct subsidies, while producers of meat, dairy, and feed crops got 73 percent![477] Between 1996 and 2005, meat subsidies reached nearly three billion dollars, and dairy product subsidies were 3.12 billion![478] Wow. It must be nice for these industries to have the USDA bailing them out whenever they have a surplus of items. What, exactly, do they do with all this food that *we* pay for? Ever hear of the National School Lunch Program (NSLP)? It's a nationwide $8 billion scheme that allows the USDA to buy up all this meat, milk, and cheese with our tax dollars and then dump this crap into the bodies of more than 28 million school children.[479] Ever wonder why school lunches are *required* to include milk? The NSLP directly benefits the meat, dairy, and poultry industries at the expense of our nation's children. In 2003, *over half* of the USDA's $41.6 billion budget was used for food assistance and nutrition programs for low-income families and children.[480]

Skinny **Bastard**

In 1999, a ground beef plant in Texas failed a series of USDA tests for salmonella. The tests showed that as much as 47 percent of the company's ground beef contained salmonella—a proportion 5 times higher than what USDA regulations allow. Despite this and the fact that high levels of salmonella in ground beef indicate high levels of fecal contamination, the USDA continued to purchase thousands of tons of the meat for distribution in schools. In fact, this company was one of the nation's largest suppliers for the school meals, providing as much as 45 percent of the program's ground meat.[481]

Contamination aside, according to Michele Simon of the Center for Informed Food Choices, "One evaluation of the commodity foods program estimates that 70 percent of the items offered exceed the U.S. dietary guidelines for fat."[482] For decades, consumer advocacy groups have been horrified by this unhealthy, profit-driven arrangement. With the backing of countless parents, physicians, and nutritionists, they have battled to get soy milk and other healthier choices approved by the USDA for use in school lunches. But the USDA (aka the beef, pork, poultry, and dairy industries) wants no part in this, of course.

The USDA has fifteen food assistance programs, including ones for the elderly, homeless, military, and poor. It is estimated that one in five Americans will take part in this $53 billion program.[483] Sounds like the USDA is helping to feed a lot of people, right? Right. They are feeding them fattening, unhealthy, artery-clogging, heart-stopping, acid-producing, contaminated meat, poultry, and dairy—with our money. How generous.

Organic or Not?

It's not enough that they dictate all things meat and dairy, the USDA even sticks its big nose into our organic products, too. In April 2004, the USDA made sweeping changes to its National Organic Program (NOP) standards. The new rules infuriated organic farmers and consumers because: livestock were allowed to eat nonorganic fishmeal, even if it contained toxins or synthetic preservatives; cows and calves given growth hormones, antibiotics, or other drugs could still provide the public with "organic" milk as long as a year had passed since the drugs were administered; pesticides could be used even if they contained unknown inert ingredients as long as a "reasonable effort" had been made to identify them; and seafood, pet food, clothing, fertilizers, and body care products could be labeled organic without being monitored by the USDA.[484] Not only were people livid with the actual changes but also with the decision-making process. By law, these types of regulatory changes are required to undergo a period of public comment before being enacted. There was no comment period, just an announcement of changes after the fact.[485]

According to Ronnie Cummins, national director of Organic Consumers Association (OCA), "Rather than comply with regulations which uphold the integrity of organic food, corporate-run factory farms, who want a piece of the $11 billion a year organic industry, are manipulating the USDA and Congress to change the rules to suit their toxic-industrial style of farming. Allowing nonorganic and potentially genetically engineered feed to be included under the definition of organic is a major setback for the integrity of what is the fastest grow-ing sector of the food industry in this country."[486] Thanks to the phone calls, letters, e-mails, and faxes of many pissed-off consumers, the USDA reversed all these changes in May 2004.[487]

Even so, many people are still mistrustful of the USDA. The non-profit group Center for Food Safety (CFS) claims that the USDA may be allowing "sham" certifiers under the umbrella of the NOP.

Have No Faith

Their suspicions were aroused by the high volume of certifications issued within a short time. These worries were heightened when the USDA refused to provide CFS with requested documents, even though they were required to do so under the Freedom of Information Act.[488]

Other environmental groups along with the OCA have joined a lawsuit against the USDA. Among their complaints is the fact that the USDA's NOP created an additional category of certified products, which directly opposes legislation put in place by Congress. They state, "When Congress has spoken clearly on a subject, USDA has no discretion to rewrite the statute making exceptions that dilute the standards of the Act."[489] Can you believe the nerve of these USDA fuckers? Going against laws created by our elected officials and making up their own rules? It's fucking mutiny is what it is. Trust no one.

Surely you've seen the "organic" Horizon brand of dairy products in your grocery store? It is the nation's largest supplier of organic dairy products. Well, it just so happens that Horizon has been accused of violating organic standards. The Cornucopia Institute, a watchdog group in support of organic agriculture, filed two complaints with the USDA. They allege that two major farms that supply Horizon with milk are confining cows in an industrial setting and denying them access to pasture, yet are still calling their products organic.[490]

Why is all this allowed to happen? Don't our elected officials know what's going on? Why don't they try to stop this? Some do. But many politicians are in bed with the evil industries. In 2000, more than $34 million was made in campaign contributions.[491] Hate to sound like a broken record, but trust no one.

Is Everyone in the FDA on Drugs?

This greed-induced immorality isn't applicable just to Congress or the USDA. The Food and Drug Administration is a pathetic facade, too. In 1990, the Monsanto Company sought FDA approval for Posilac, a commercialized form of bovine growth hormone (BGH, used to increase cows' milk production). Even though the test study linked the hormone to prostate and thyroid cancer, the FDA approved Posilac. Of course, these damning test results weren't made available to the public until 1998, when a group of scientists conducted an independent analysis of the study. They found that the FDA never even reviewed Monsanto's findings! More recently, BGH has been linked to increased levels of Insulin Growth Factor-1, a cancer promoter. But the FDA has no interest in these findings, either. Or the fact that both the World Trade Organization and The United Nations Food Standards Body refuse to endorse the hormone's safety. And they certainly don't mind that BGH milk is banned in all of the European Union, Canada, Japan, and every other industrialized country in the world.[492] Fucking dumbasses.

Why would the FDA knowingly allow a cancer-causing hormone into our milk supply? One theory highlights the fact that the FDA deputy commissioner at the time of the Posilac approval was a former Monsanto lawyer. And during his tenure at the FDA, this same deputy commissioner wrote the policy exempting BGH from special labeling. Yet, fingers also point to a former top scientist with Monsanto, who was hired by the FDA to review her own research, conducted while she was working for Monsanto. This little beauty also allowed a hundredfold increase of antibiotic residues in milk.[493]

The FDA's bad behavior isn't singular to the dairy industry. It also has a sketchy history with monosodium glutamate (MSG). One former FDA commissioner testified before the Senate Select Committee on Nutrition that MSG was safe, citing four sources. It was later discovered that two of the studies were nonexistent, and the other two were incomplete![494]

Secrets and lies. It's just too much to bear. So let's also play the "I'm not telling" game. Ever see the words "natural flavors" on food packaging ingredient lists? Yeah, that's because the FDA allows companies to be vague and doesn't require them to tell us exactly what we're eating. The FDA has a list of approximately 300 foods that meet a "standard of identity," meaning companies aren't required to spell out their ingredients. For example, ice cream manufacturers can use any of twenty-five specified additives without listing them in their ingredients.[495] Who wants to put something into his or her body without even knowing what it is?

You Are Your Only Chance

If you want to get healthy/buff, you can rely on only yourself. If you adapt only one practice from this book, let it be this: *Read the ingredients.* Forget counting carbs, adding calories, and multiplying fat grams. Just read the ingredients. It doesn't matter how many calories or carbs or fat grams something has. You don't need the government's asinine recommended daily allowances to tell you how to eat. Just read the ingredients. If they are healthy, wholesome, and pure—dive in. If there is refined sugar, white or bleached flour, hydrogenated oils, any animal products, artificial anything, or some scary looking word that you don't know—don't eat it. We can't make it any simpler. Just read the ingredients and completely ignore all the other gibber-jabber bullshit the government calls for on the packaging. Fuck them. Trust no one. Get ripped.

And no matter what, do not fall prey to clever adjectives used on the packaging. The companies that call their products "wholesome" or "nutritious" can be the same ones that add hydrogenated oils, artificial flavors, or synthetic preservatives. Just read the ingredients of everything you buy. It's not a big deal, assuming you are literate. There is so much bureaucracy and red tape surrounding health-related government agencies that you are much better off fending for yourself. After all, why would anyone take nutritional advice from organizations that let color dyes, hydrogenated oils, chemical preservatives, and artificial flavors into the food we eat?

The EPA Makes Us Sick

StarLink corn, a genetically modified organism, contains an insecticidal protein deemed unsafe for human consumption. But the Environmental Protection Agency allows the use of StarLink for livestock feed.[496] Let humans eat the animals who ate the corn? That's safe? Duh.

Clearly, nothing is sacred to the group that allows *rocket fuel* in our milk supply. Yeah, you heard right. Rocket fuel. In milk. Thanks to the Pentagon, ammonium perchlorate, the main explosive component in rocket fuel, has been lurking around our environment for decades. It finds its way into water used for growing feed crops for cattle. Cows eat these contaminated crops, resulting in contaminated milk. Whether you are drinking milk or eating dairy products made with this milk, you are ingesting perchlorate. And the EPA actually makes allowances for a "provisional daily safe dose."[497] We're sorry, but where we're from— Earth—there is no acceptable amount to ingest where explosive components are concerned. Even if you believe any amount to be safe, tests revealed milk perchlorate levels well above the EPA's index. Studies conducted by the Environmental Working Group (EWG), a nonprofit, nonpartisan organization, found *every single* milk sample tested in Texas to be contaminated. California's own Food and Agriculture Department found that milk off the grocers' shelves had *five* times the EPA's "safe dose" of perchlorate. But, of course, the California Food and Agriculture Department did not release these results. Instead, they were brought to light by the EWG. Although both the dairy industry and government agencies acknowledge that there could be some health risks associated with perchlorate, they maintain that we should keep drinking milk for its "calcium, protein, and minerals."[498] We'll let you use your own heads on this one.

Regardless of your political affiliation, please know this: The Bush Administration continuously asked for exemptions on behalf of the military and chemical companies, allowing them to continue this contamination and to shirk responsibility for cleanup. In fact, the Bush administration's EPA was widely criticized on many counts of environmental pollution that affect our food and water supply. Like the USDA's pathetic voluntary program, the EPA has its own version of letting agribusiness trample all over public health and safety. Collaborating closely with the U.S. Poultry and Egg Association and the National Pork Producers Council (NPPC), the EPA developed a *voluntary* air-monitoring program. Disregard the notion that the EPA blames factory farming for 73 percent of all ammonia (fumes from all the shit and piss of farm animals) released into the air nationwide. Never mind the fact that the EPA names factory farming to be the single largest contributor of polluted American waterways. Factory farmers do not have to submit to EPA monitoring programs.[499] If it pleases them, they can volunteer. How civilized.

Outraged by the EPA's lack of enforcement, opponents point out that the factory farming industry made $3.46 million in campaign contributions, benefiting mostly Republican federal candidates. The NPPC even went so far as to present President Bush with its "Friend of the Pork Producer" award in 2004, thanking him for his help in "shaping environmental policies impacting agriculture."[500] Yeah, um, thanks for that.

Trust No One

Whether you love him or hate him, President Clinton's administration tried to "implement a tough, science-based food inspection system," according to Eric Schlosser, bestselling author of *Fast Food Nation*. Sad to say, however, these attempts were squashed when the

Have No Faith

Republican party gained control of Congress in 1994. Schlosser revealed, "The meatpacking industry's allies in Congress worked hard to thwart modernization of the nation's meat inspection system. A great deal of effort was spent denying the federal government any authority to recall contaminated meat or impose civil fines on firms that knowingly ship contaminated products. . . . The Clinton Administration backed legislation to provide the USDA with the authority to demand meat recalls and impose civil fines on meatpackers. [But] Republicans in Congress failed to enact not only that bill, but also similar legislation [for four consecutive years]. . . . Under current law, the USDA cannot demand a recall [of contaminated meat]." Can you fucking believe this? If a company decides voluntarily to recall contaminated meat, "it is under no legal obligation to inform the public—or even health officials—that a recall is taking place."[501]

Now, we don't mean to say that everyone working for the government is evil. There are some decent, caring, moral, intelligent, well-intentioned people working for the FDA, EPA, and USDA. One former staff attorney-turned-environmentalist said the EPA "hasn't initiated one investigation in four years. They're not doing anything."[502]

See, she's a "good guy"! She finked on the EPA. Unfortunately, however, the majority of good guys seem to be lost in the shuffle of politics and greed within these groups.

So do yourself a favor and trust no one. Read ingredients. Ignore everything else. And, if you're totally incensed by what you've just learned, do something. Contact your representatives, senators, the president, and vice president, and demand reform of these crooked, self-serving agencies. Go to www.congress.org to send a quick e-mail to these politicians. While you're at it, write a letter to the editor of your favorite magazine or newspaper and ask others to join the crusade. Visit www.congress.org and click on the "media guide" to access their contact information.

Chapter 11

Don't Be a Pussy

What if someone told you you that you could totally change your life and have the body you want for the rest of your life? What if all you had to do was follow a simple formula and maybe struggle for a month or two? What if you could reprogram your brain to actually enjoy healthy foods? Well, guess what? You *can* change your life. You *can* have the body you want for the *rest of your life*. You can enjoy healthy foods. All you have to do is follow a simple formula and be willing to delay gratification for a few months. A few months. That's it. Then you can enjoy a new body for the rest of your life. Don't be a pussy. You have all the nutritional information you need to become a Skinny Bastard. The rest is up to you. Although this is a lifestyle and not a diet, it is going to feel like a diet for the first thirty days or so. During this time, you will be retraining your brain, healing your taste buds, and cleansing and detoxifying your body. It might suck a little. Chances are there will be times you feel deprived, angry, overwhelmed, and frustrated. But these few, fleeting moments will all be worthwhile once you are buff. Truth be told, if you follow our guidelines, it won't be so bad.

Before you even start making changes, take notice of how you feel and the role that your diet plays. Do you wake up tired? Is coffee the only thing that gets you going in the morning? Are you cranky in the afternoon? Do you need snacks to bolster your mood? Do you have little or no energy? Do you rely on soda or sugar for a little boost? Do you have trouble falling asleep? Is a beer (or three) the only thing that gets you drowsy? When you eat something unhealthy, how do you feel while you're eating it? Right after? An hour later? How does it affect your sleep that night? How do you feel the next day? Pay attention to the negative effects your current diet and lifestyle have on your body, moods, and energy level. If it's not too girlie, feel free to start a little journal, writing what you eat and drink throughout the day and how you feel as a result. This way, when you start making positive changes to your diet, you'll appreciate all of the results—not just the weight loss.

Recognize that anything worth having is worth fighting for. Good

Don't Be a Pussy

health, vitality, more energy, more confidence, better sex, great abs—
you either want 'em or you don't. You can continue plodding along in
your life feeling like you're not living up to your man potential or you
can dedicate yourself to creating the life you want. Fuck excuses about
not having the time. You spend at least forty hours a week working.
And fuck excuses about it being "too hard" to eat well. Certainly your
health and your body are more important than anything else in your
life. You are worthless to your company, colleagues, friends, and family if you do not value yourself enough to take excellent care of
yourself. Love yourself enough to do whatever it takes to be the best
you you can be.

An important part of any recovery program for addiction—and
unhealthy eating is an addiction—is taking it one day at a time. Don't
torture yourself with thoughts of "I can never eat steak again" or
"How will I live without coffee?" Just take it one meal at a time. Don't
think ahead with dread and anguish. One meal at a time. And when all
feels hopeless, remember that you are in charge of what goes into your
body, you don't answer to anyone, and you are *allowed* to eat anything
you want. Often just knowing we *can* eat whatever we want is enough
to keep us from eating whatever we want. We're so rebellious.

If you feel really invigorated and motivated and you're ready to completely immerse yourself in the Skinny Bastard lifestyle now, then rock on. Go for it. Otherwise, feel free to set mini-goals for yourself and tackle them one at a time. This means spend the first week of your new life removing one dirty vice item. Whether it's cigarettes or coffee or alcohol or sugar or junk food or meat or dairy—just purge something negative from your life immediately. Choose something that you like and enjoy but that you know you can let go of successfully. (But start right now. Don't let these intense feelings fade—use them.) Dedicate the week to getting this vice item out of your diet, your body, your kitchen, and your mind. Think of all you've learned about this item and how disgusting it is. Envision the damaging effect it has on your organs, your moods, your health, and your appearance. Imagine exactly what it is that you'd be eating. Know how shitty you'd feel, physically and mentally, if you ate it. Understand that you have free will and that if you *wanted* to eat it, you could. But know with every fiber and cell of your being that *today* you wish to put only pure, beautiful, healthful foods in your body. Most important, acknowledge that no vice item will ever make you feel happy or whole or satisfied. In fact, all vice items make you *unhappy* because they contribute to weight issues, health problems, mood swings, and low self-esteem.

When you've got one week under your belt, feel great about what you've accomplished. Then, immediately, while continuing to steer clear of the item you banished in Week One, start Week Two by ridding something else from your diet. Every week, until you've completely cleansed your life of poison and toxins, eliminate one more thing. Apply the same mindset, dedication, technique, and excitement you used in Week One. Resign yourself to purifying your thoughts, body, and kitchen of this crappy vice item; realize you've just made your life better by not letting this item infect you anymore; gross yourself out thinking about what exactly it is and the effects it has on your body; think of how bad it makes you feel when you partake in it; and finally, remember that if you did *choose* to eat/smoke/drink it, it wouldn't make you happy or fulfilled.

Never feel like or say you are "giving up" your favorite foods. Those words have a negative connotation, like you are sacrificing something. You're not *giving up* anything. You are simply empowered now and able to make educated, controlled choices about what you will and won't put into your body, your temple. Be grateful that you now know the truth about the foods you used to poison yourself with.

Let all you think and speak of regarding this life change be positive. People who have positive attitudes are much more successful than those who don't. Be excited about feeling clean, pure, healthy, energized, happy, and buff. Enjoy every second of this metamorphosis, knowing the journey is as important as the end result.

Confucius never said, "A hungry man is a bratty, babyish asshole," but he should have. Because it's true. A hungry man is a wah-wah crybaby, who will destroy everything and everyone in his path if hunger is allowed to set in. So you must always be prepared with healthy food on hand. Otherwise, seriously, you will fall off the wagon almost immediately. Your kitchen should be stocked at all times with the appropriate foods. Pack your lunch and a snack for school or work. Keep an emergency stash in your car, at your desk, and in your murse (man-purse). Never, ever get caught with your pants down. Unfortunately, depending on where you live, restaurants may not be a safe place for the first month. The menu might not have any vegan or even vegetarian options, and it is easy to be hypnotized by the seductive smells of cooking. This doesn't mean you can't eat out ever again as long as you live. Just for thirty days. (Unless there are good veggie-friendly restaurants in your neighborhood. Asian, Mexican, and Italian restaurants almost always have veggie choices.) You can't expect to change your life without a few minor adjustments. Your only priority for thirty days is to adhere to the regimen you're creating. Without straying. After you achieve thirty days of pure eating, you'll feel confident you have what it takes to get the job done. "I just survived thirty days. I'm so proud of myself. This is the healthiest I've ever been in my whole life. If I *want* to, I can eat an old vice item. But why would I? I just made it thirty consecutive days. I'm going to keep going." If you test yourself before thirty days, you are setting yourself up for failure. Be patient and strong.

When you reach the thirty-day milestone, don't run out and gorge yourself on crap. In fact, just keep doing what you've been doing. See and feel all the positive changes in your body, energy level, and self-esteem. Alcohol, cigarettes, coffee, and food are all addictive, physically and psychologically. Chances are, even after the thirty days, if you indulge in a vice item, you might go off the deep end. It is well known in Alcoholics Anonymous that you're only "one drink away from your next drunk." This means we think we can control our addictions. "I'll just have one drink. I'll just have pizza this one time. I'll just eat half a piece of cake." The truth of the matter is that we are powerless over our addictions. We don't want to make you feel like you can never eat your favorite foods ever again. We just want to impress upon you that it is very easy to obliterate all your progress with one bite, sip, or puff.

After one month of pure living, if you did eat the food you've been fantasizing about, you probably wouldn't even enjoy it. Really. You'd see that your brain has been tricking you and your taste buds all along. Now that your taste buds have healed and become more sensitized and your brain knows the truth, those old chemical, sugary, artificial, dead, rotting foods will taste "off" or "less than" somehow.

If you do decide to partake in a vice item after thirty days, it cannot be out of weakness or for lack of preparation. You should never be somewhere and just say, "Fuck it." It should be a calculated, scheduled, premeditated choice. The portion should be decided on beforehand, should be smaller than you would normally have had, and served on a plate. (The package should be put away before you start eating.) Sit down at a table. Eat very slowly. Try not to finish the whole thing. Do not have another serving. Take note of how you feel while you're eating it, immediately after, an hour later, in bed that night, and the next day. Chances are, because your body is now pure, the vice item will make you feel a little nauseated or headache-y at the very least. And it most certainly won't taste as good as you imagine it will. Do not discount these negative feelings. They are your new, healthy, clean, pure organs speaking to you.

Enough of all this melodrama. It's not like you're gonna be hungry and cranky for all of eternity. We know that dieters always "crash" when their favorite foods become forbidden. So we devised the *Skinny Bastard* plan to allow for cookies, cakes, chocolate, burgers, ice cream, etc. They just aren't the same ones you're used to. You're not giving up anything; you're just trading in all your old, gross food. Big deal. The new stuff is just as good. So don't kid yourself with the old "I had a craving" routine. Nobody's buying it.

The only thing more annoying than the "Where do you get your protein?" question is the "My body is craving meat, I must need protein" comment. Most cravings are not reliable indicators of what your body needs. Smokers crave cigarettes, alcoholics crave alcohol, drug addicts crave drugs, and junk food eaters crave junk. If you eat shit for a few days and you begin to crave a salad or a piece of fruit, that's a craving you can trust. Otherwise, it's just your addiction talking. Bitch-slap it and get a hold of yourself. But feel free to try and understand your addiction first.

For us to survive, our brains came equipped with dopamine, a pleasure-producing chemical. Dopamine is released during sex (or even just while flirting) so that we'll procreate and the human race won't die out. And food stimulates dopamine release so that we'll remember to eat and nourish our bodies. Basically, anything the brain perceives as enjoyable will cause dopamine to lock onto brain cells and build a permanent memory trace of where pleasure comes from.[503] Even though this evolved out of the need for survival, sometimes it can be a bad thing. Heroin, cocaine, alcohol, and nicotine all trigger the brain's pleasure circuitry. And not surprisingly, chocolate, sugar, and cheese affect this same part of the brain.[504] So you see, we can be *physiologically* addicted to food. Any food can trigger the brain's pleasure center. Some of us are fortunate enough to experience dopamine ecstasy while eating broccoli, and we actually crave this healthy food. But the types of food and the degree of pleasure they bring will differ from one person to the next. The trick is resetting our memory traces to feel pleasure from healthy food and no pleasure from junk food.[505]

Easier said than done. Especially for people who are addicted to cigarettes, alcohol, or drugs or who are overweight. Studies have shown that these people have fewer receptors for dopamine than other people. For them, the pleasure-giving chemical has fewer places to attach to brain cells, making it difficult for them to experience pleasurable feelings. So, because they aren't getting that "pleasure rush," they tend to smoke, drink, use drugs, gamble, or overeat.[506] Now don't automatically diagnose yourself as one these people and assume you'll never get healthy. We are not at the mercy of our bodies. We are the commanders of our bodies.[507]

Unless we eat cheese. Cheese will rule our lives and fatten our asses if we don't kick the addiction. Cow's milk actually has traces of morphine in it![508] And for once, we can't blame factory farming. Morphine, along with codeine and other opiates, are naturally produced in cows' livers and end up in their milk.[509] But that's not all. All milk, whether from a cow or a human, contains *casein*, a protein that breaks apart during digestion and releases a whole slew of opiates. All these "feel good" chemicals exist so that newborns will nurse and thrive and to ensure a bond between mothers and their young.[510]

Are you starting to get the picture? When a woman breastfeeds, her milk has an almost drug-like effect on the baby. The baby is totally hooked. He'll cry, not because he's hungry, but because he needs "a fix" of that pleasurable feeling produced by the opiates. Nature has guaranteed that our babies will nurse and grow. And when they reach a certain age, we wean them and stop giving them these "drugs." And they're fine. But then we start them on cows' milk and an addiction is born.

All dairy products contain casein, but cheese has the highest concentration.[511] In fact, cheese contains far more casein than is naturally found in cows' milk. It also has phenylethylamine, an amphetamine-like chemical.[512] So when we kid around and say, "I am addicted to cheese," it's not a joke—it's true. We are chemically addicted to cheese.[513]

Casein even finds its way into soy cheese. Whether manufacturers use it to up the protein content, to aid in melting, or because they know of its addictive quality, casein still has the same effect. So if you see casein on the list of ingredients, run! (Follow Your Heart cheeses are casein-free and totally vegan, so enjoy.)

The following hormones and natural chemicals have all been identified in cows' milk: prolactin, somatostatin, melatonin, oxytocin, growth hormone, leuteinizing hormone-releasing hormone, thyrotropin-releasing hormone, thyroid-stimulating hormone, vasoactive intestinal peptide, calcitonin, parathyroid hormone, corticosteroids, estrogens, progesterone, insulin, epidermal growth factor, insulin-like growth factor, erythropoietin, bombesin, neurotensin, motilin, and cholecystokinin.[514] If you think your will is strong enough to conquer all those motherfuckers, you're on drugs! Dairy is fattening,[515] and if you eat it, you'll never find your abs. You cannot control your addiction. You can't "just have one slice of pizza" or "only have cheese at parties." You're "only one piece of cheese" away from a total relapse. Eat the substitutes; they'll get you through.

Thankfully, our bodies produce a few different chemical substances that help tame our appetites. One such hormone, leptin, is made by our fat cells. When fat cells in our bodies get adequate nourishment, they release leptin into the blood for two purposes.[516] The first is to alert the brain to diminish the appetite. Next, our metabolism gets boosted, encouraging the body's cells to burn calories more quickly.[517] Pretty cool, huh? Until we start "dieting." Typical low-calorie diets confuse the body into thinking it's starving. So our fat cells slow down their leptin production to help *increase* our appetites.[518] Release the hounds! Now we feel like we're starving! So we trash our diets and binge like beasts. But diets high in fat don't fare any better. Fatty diets (think animal products) also lower leptin levels. You know where this is headed: Low-fat, plant-based diets actually boost leptin levels, helping each molecule of leptin to work more effectively.[519] So help yourself succeed.

Eating healthy foods like fruits, vegetables, whole grains, and beans will help curb your appetite and stimulate your metabolism.[520]

Even if you do have some serious cravings, the good thing about the *Skinny Bastard* plan is that there are plenty of naughty-tasting foods that you don't need to feel bad about. So eat all day long. As long as everything you put in your mouth meets Skinny Bastard approval, it's fine. Just be sure that when you're full, you *stop eating*. We know this is a foreign concept, but we're hoping it'll catch on. Visualize the actual size of your stomach (about the size of a one-quart container). Imagine what size you want it to be. There is no need to cram it full and stretch the shit out of it three times a day, every day, for your entire life. Look at the portion you put on your plate. Do you think it will fit in your stomach nicely, or that you'll need to force it in? Pare down.

Just because you're "starving," you don't need to eat faster. When you're done eating, if you have the hiccups, indigestion, a stomachache, or you're burping and farting, that means you're eating too fast and gulping down air. Slow down. Breathe evenly. Conversely, make sure you aren't holding your breath. Also, be sure to chew your food purposefully and slowly. Rest in between bites. Do not watch TV, read a magazine, talk on the phone, or do *anything else* while you are eating. The goal is to know when you're full (without having *stuffed* yourself) and be able to put the fork down. You aren't six anymore. You won't get the praise of elders for cleaning your plate. It's okay to leave food on your plate.

But if you do still get off on scoring brownie points, you can earn extra credit by fasting. Yeah, fasting—willfully abstaining from food. For more than 5,000 years, fasting has been used as a healthy method of weight loss.[521] It is also a powerful tool for cleaning, flushing, detoxifying, and maintaining the body and healing illnesses, minor and major.[522] When we eat, all of our body's energy goes toward digesting, using, and storing the food and eliminating the waste. When we don't eat, all of our body's energy goes toward cleaning house. And with all the years of abuse, our house could sure use a cleaning. We absorb toxic chemicals from food, drinks, and the environment. Our body eliminates some of these through waste, but the rest remain as chemical byproducts and free radicals (highly reactive chemicals that damage cells and contribute to premature aging, heart disease, and cancer). Fasting gets rid of these toxins. It also increases our blood's white cell count, which boosts immunity and protects us from disease. And because fasting is beneficial for the circulatory system, you can expect better skin and hair.[523]

Fasts can last anywhere from twenty-four hours to ten days or more. It's all up to you and how much you need to cleanse, but even just one day once a month is beneficial. There are too many types of fasts to cover them all, so we'll explain just a few. It is imperative to really read up on fasting before diving in.

A particular favorite is a raw or "live" food fast, when, obviously, you eat only raw foods for however many days you choose. This is a great beginner's fast because you reap the benefits of fasting while still being able to actually eat. It's also a good fast to do if you want to work your way up to a more stringent fast, like a juice fast, where the only thing you put in your body is fresh-pressed or fresh-squeezed juice (not pasteurized or packaged). Whether it's fruit juice, veggie juice, or both, the enzymes are wonderful aides in the cleansing process. A liquid fast is similar to the juice fast, but includes soups, too (no beans or rice or chunks—just liquid). The alkalizing properties of the juices and soups help to neutralize the toxins being released from the body.[524] For this and other reasons, the hardest fast is a water fast, where you have nothing but water. Don't be a competitive asshole and launch yourself into this fast from the diet you exist on now. You've gotta learn to

Don't Be a Pussy

crawl before you can walk.

Most people like to ease into a fast. They might eat smaller portions for a week prior. Or if they usually eat vegan junk food, they might abstain in preparation. We highly recommend eating as purely as possible a week or two leading up to a fast. (Meat-eaters should go vegetarian and then vegan before fasting.) It makes the transition more gradual and less jarring. Regardless of which fast you choose, be sure to drink a lot of water throughout. Your body will be detoxing like crazy, and you don't want to become dehydrated.

All fasts are challenging, both physically and mentally. Do not expect it to be easy, especially at the beginning when you find yourself salivating over foods you don't normally even care about. But eventually, you get to a place where you are truly not hungry, and you feel light, clean, clear, and almost divine. When you do reintroduce food back into your diet, which should be done slowly, with great care, you are almost repulsed by things you previously ate. It is quite beautiful to have such a new, fresh perspective. Periodic repeated fasts are especially useful for this reason. They help our bodies and minds establish a new relationship with food. In fact, because of this, fasting can even be used to overcome addictions. When we eliminate the toxins that cause "cell memory cravings," we can eradicate the need for the food or drug that provided those toxins.[525]

Not surprisingly, some people experience headaches, weakness, nausea, cramping, stomach pains, sweating, a swollen tongue, bad breath, general aches and pains, increased temperature, or depression while fasting.[526] Abstaining from food does not *cause* these ailments. They are simply normal side effects of fasting. After two to three days of fasting, the body goes into autolysis and actually starts digesting its own cells. With its wisdom, the body selectively decomposes the tissues and cells that are in excess (fat), diseased, damaged, old, or dead.[527] The body is literally digesting and expelling poisons, toxins, and bad cells that were already there—and it feels crappy. This is actually a good thing, because the body is finally able to tackle some problems that were lurking within.

During a fast, digestive enzymes are relieved from their usual role and instead act to cleanse and rejuvenate the body. This rejuvenation process includes the production of new cells. And when more cells are being produced than are dying, the aging process is actually being reversed.[528] This phenomenon occurs during juice and water fasts. Eventually, you'll notice sharper senses of smell, sight, sound, and taste. You'll feel lighter physically, mentally, and emotionally.[529]

All magic aside, fasting is *not* for you if you're underweight or suffering from severe wasting diseases, such as neurological degenerative diseases and certain cancers. Diabetics and people suffering from hypoglycemia can fast, but only with medical supervision.[530] For that matter, anyone with any medical condition should consult his doctor before fasting.

Vitamins are an integral part of a healthy lifestyle. Here are some significant vitamins and minerals, a description of why they're important, and which foods provide them. (Warning: this section is kinda boring.)

Calcium strengthens bones, provides for healthy teeth, reduces risk of colon cancer, decreases chances of bone loss, aids the nervous system, and alleviates insomnia. Eat almonds, Brazil and other nuts, seeds, soybeans, kale, collard greens, broccoli, kelp, blackstrap molasses, and calcium-fortified soy or hemp milk to get calcium.

Folic acid promotes healthy skin, protects against parasites and food poisoning, and helps ward off anemia. To get folic acid, eat leafy green veggies, carrots, artichokes, fruit, cantaloupe, avocados, apricots, beans, lentils, soybeans, garbanzo beans, barley, and whole wheat.

Iron aids growth, promotes resistance to disease, prevents fatigue and anemia, and enhances good skin tone. It can be found in nuts, pumpkin seeds, beans, lentils, whole grains, oatmeal, asparagus, molasses, and seaweed.

Magnesium (known as the anti-stress mineral) fights depression, boosts energy, helps burn fat, prevents heart attacks, maintains good cholesterol levels, aids indigestion, and keeps teeth strong and healthy. When combined with calcium, it works as a natural tranquilizer. Eat nuts, seeds, sunflower seeds, green vegetables, soybeans, kelp (seaweed), and molasses to get a good dose.

Omega-3 fatty acids fight heart disease, lower bad cholesterol levels, help fight depression, lessen the likelihood of blood clots, reduce the risk of breast cancer, help with rheumatoid arthritis, and keep skin, hair, and nails healthy. (You know you care.) Sources for these fatty acids are flaxseeds, walnuts, soybeans, pumpkin seeds, canola oil, and hempseeds and their oil.

Potassium aids in reducing blood pressure, increases clear thinking by helping send oxygen to the brain, and helps the body dispose of waste. It's found in bananas, citrus fruits, cantaloupe, tomatoes, watercress, green leafy vegetables, sunflower seeds, avocados, lentils, potatoes, and whole grains.

B vitamins improve mental attitude, aid in digestion, help migraine headaches, contribute to healthy skin, act as natural diuretics, strengthen immunity, increase energy, improve concentration and memory, and are good for the nervous system. Eat whole wheat, wheat germ, bran, oatmeal, whole grains, brown rice, beans, nuts, seeds, soybeans, lentils, dates, figs, bananas, and vegetables.

Vitamin C accelerates healing, lowers blood pressure, prevents colds, protects against cancer, and helps decrease blood cholesterol. It also forms collagen, which is important for growth, repair, tissue cells, blood vessels, gums, bones, and teeth. It's easy to get vitamin C by eating broccoli, Brussels sprouts, cabbage, collard greens, green peppers, spinach, watercress, potatoes, grapefruits, oranges, and papayas.

Vitamin D, in conjunction with calcium and phosphorous, helps build strong bones and teeth. Not only does vitamin D help our bodies assimilate vitamin A, but it also prevents colds when teamed up with vitamins A and C. Vitamin D can be obtained from getting direct sun on the skin or from supplements.

Vitamin E keeps you looking younger, inhibits cancer cell growth, fights fatigue, prevents blood clots, lowers blood pressure, decreases the risk of Alzheimer's disease, and accelerates the healing of burns. It's found in wheat germ, whole-grain cereals, whole wheat, nuts, sunflower seeds, leafy greens, and vegetable oils.

Zinc helps with infertility issues, is important for brain function, maintains the body's acid/alkaline balance, aids in collagen formation, and helps form insulin (needed for many vital enzymes). Foods with high concentrations of zinc are wheat germ, whole grains, pumpkin seeds, sesame seeds, and soybeans.[531]

When we eat properly, we can get almost all of the nutrients we need from food sources; however, all vegans and vegetarians should supplement with vitamins B-12 and D, as well as omega-3 fatty acids. B-12 is made in the intestines of animals (even human animals), but we need more than what we make.[532] Research has shown that plants grown in high-quality soil have a good concentration of readily absorbable B-12.[533] But sadly, nowadays, the soil quality has been depleted and compromised with poor farming methods and the use of all the pesticides and chemicals, and our plant foods may not supply us with adequate amounts of B-12.[534]

Research of late has found that vitamin D deficiency is a big problem—not only for vegetarians, but for everyone.[535] Vitamin D is in short supply in our food (even "good" sources, such as fish, may not be so great after all), and while sun exposure is the most common way to get D, it's not enough for most.[536] If you live north of Atlanta, you're getting essentially no D during the winter. And if you wear sunscreen during summer, you can kiss the D goodbye all year long.[537] Good vitamin D status protects us against a slew of diseases, including heart disease and cancer.[538] Experts are recommending that we all take 1,000 International Units a day.[539]

The omega-3s, again, are important for brain function, behavioral issues, and protection from chronic disease,[540] and as we mentioned they can be found in whole grains, beans, seaweed, and soybean products.[541] Some people think that eating fish is a good source, but they're also getting all the contaminants and toxic pollutants that were absorbed into the fish's flesh.[542] So instead, you can get your omega-3's from the same source the fish gets it—microalgae, tiny sea plants.[543] Luckily, you don't have to go trolling the ocean floor; DHA microalgae supplements are available, and they, along with good plant sources of omega-3, will ensure a healthy supply. If you can't find them in your local health store, get 'em online at Vegetarianvitamin.com (Deva Vegan Omega-3 DHA softgels) or Veganessentials.com (Udo's DHA Oil Blend or O-mega-Zen3 Liquid Vegan DHA Supplement by NuTru). Pop a cap a day.

Keep in mind that a healthy balance of fatty acids isn't only about getting your 3s but about going easy on the omega-6s, which most of us get too much of.[544] So maximize the foods high in omega 3s but at the same time, pass up the fried foods, fast food, high-fat snacks, and convenience foods, which are heavy on the 6s.[545] Enjoy high mono fats too, like what you'll get in olive oil and avocados, for an optimal balance of fats.[546]

Chapter 12

Soup's On

We *truly* want to help you succeed and make this all as easy as possible. In this chapter, we've compiled a few lists so that there will be no confusion as to what you should or shouldn't eat. After reading the whole book, if you're feeling uncertain about what to buy or order, just whip out your *Skinny Bastard* and come right to this chapter. There will be no doubt that you're making the right food choices.

Breakfast is the most important meal of the day. But not why you think. The cereal and dairy industries lead us to believe that without a big, "healthy" breakfast, we won't have enough energy to get us through the day. But Sugar Smacks with cow's milk hardly constitutes a healthy, viable energy source. The *real* reason breakfast is so important is that it sets the tone for your entire day of eating. If you eat a shitty breakfast, you will likely crave (and eat) crap all day. And if you eat too early in the morning, you'll be interrupting your body's cleaning session. Remember, when your body isn't working on food, it's working on you! When your "cleaning crew" is in the middle of cleanup and you start cramming food in, "they" get overwhelmed. They stop what they're doing, throw their hands up, scratch their heads, and finally decide that they just can't deal with this mess you're making. So they opt to store it away as fat and pretend they'll get to it later.[547] So when you wake up, you should wait to eat breakfast until you're actually hungry. Don't just eat right away because that's what you're used to. After a few days, you'll get used to that empty feeling in your stomach and know that the initial headaches, nausea, and hunger were just your body's cleaning crew. Feel free to enjoy a cup of caffeine-free, organic, herbal tea upon waking, or a tall glass of water. But other than that, the best thing to do is wait until you're actually hungry.

When you do eat, the breakfast of Skinny Bastards always starts with fruit. Most men do not eat enough fruit. The best way to make sure you're getting enough is to get it over with first thing. After you get your fruit on, eat some healthy cereal; a whole-grain muffin, bagel, or toast; or get fancy and whip up some tofu scramble, pancakes, or something else. If you need help with some product names, here are some other breakfast food suggestions:

Breakfast Food List

(R) found in refrigerator section (F) found in freezer section

Arrowhead Mills: organic blue corn pancake and waffle mix

Arrowhead Mills: organic whole-grain pancake and waffle mix

Food For Life: Ezekiel 4:9 cereal

Barbara's Bakery: Puffins cereal

Barbara's Bakery: Shredded Spoonfuls cereal

Peace Cereal: vanilla almond crisp

Peace Cereal: maple pecan crisp

Nature's Path: Optimum Slim cereal

Nature's Path: Optimum Power Breakfast cereal

Health Valley: organic raisin bran flakes

Health Valley: organic oat bran flakes with raisins

Old Wessex Ltd.: Irish-style oatmeal

Old Wessex Ltd.: 5-grain cereal

Nature's Path: organic instant hot maple nut oatmeal

Ancient Harvest: organic quinoa flakes

Rice Dream: original enriched rice milk

Original EdenSoy: organic soymilk

Original EdenBlend: rice & soy beverage

House: tofu steak (R)

Whole Soy & Co.: creamy cultured soy (yogurt) (R)

Silk: cultured soy (yogurt) (R)

Amy's: organic tofu scramble (F)

Van's: all-natural organic original waffles (F)

Lifestream: Mesa Sunrise toaster waffles

French Meadow Bakery: men's bread

French Meadow Bakery: healthy hemp sprouted bread

French Meadow Bakery: brown rice bread

Nature's Path: organic Manna breads (F)

Fabe's All Natural Bakery: vegan muffins (F)

Zen Bakery: muffins (R)

Zen Bakery: cinnamon raisin rolls (R)

Whole Foods: organic English muffins (R)

Food For Life: Ezekiel 4:9 sprouted grain bagels (F)

Tofutti: Better Than Cream Cheese (R) (the kind without hydrogenated oils)

Lightlife: Smart Bacon (R)

Lightlife: Gimme Lean! sausage style (R)

organic fruit

Lunch Food List

Don't eat lunch until you're truly hungry. This will allow your breakfast to pass through your body without having food piled on top of it. In a perfect world, lunch always includes a fresh, organic salad with lots of raw vegetables. You can build from there with the usual stuff: sandwiches, burritos, soup, baked potatoes, Chinese, Japanese, Thai, Italian, veggie burgers, soy chicken, etc. Also, here's our yummy lunch product list if you need a boost:

Food For Life: Ezekiel 4:9 bread (F) (or bakery/bread aisle)

Arrowhead Mills: organic Valencia peanut butter

MaraNatha: organic raw almond butter

Bionaturae: organic fruit spreads

Natural Touch: Tuno (faux tuna)

Morningstar Farms: Tuno

Amy's: All-American burger (F)

Amy's: California burger (F)

Amy's: Texas burger (F)

Gardenburger: flame-grilled burgers (F)

Gardenburger: flame-grilled chik'n (F)

Whole Foods Bakehouse: organic burger buns

Skinny **Bastard**

Tofurkey: deli slices

Yves: veggie bologna (R)

Yves: veggie turkey (R)

Yves: veggie salami (R)

Follow Your Heart: vegan gourmet cheese alternative (R)

Earthbound Farm: organic salad greens (R)

Fantastic Foods: tabouli

Fantastic Foods: organic whole wheat couscous

Fantastic Carb 'Tastic Soup: vegetarian chicken gumbo

Fantastic Carb 'Tastic Soup: shiitake mushroom

Fantastic Big Soup: five bean

Fantastic Big Soup: country lentil

Amy's Organic Soups: black bean vegetable

Amy's Organic Soups: butternut squash

Amy's Organic Soups: lentil vegetable

Amy's Organic Soups: chunky vegetable

Amy's: organic chili

Health Valley: organic split-pea soup

Health Valley: organic lentil soup

Health Valley: organic black bean soup

Imagine: organic vegetable broth

Soup's On

Imagine: organic no-chicken broth

Pacific: organic vegetable broth

organic vegetables

Dinner Food List

When you're feeling really hungry, it's time for din-din. Dinner is easy and fun. Just pick from the list, or create your own healthy vegan fest:

Health Best 100% Organic: red lentils

Health Best 100% Organic: green lentils

Health Best 100% Organic: barley

Health Best 100% Organic: split peas

Health Best 100% Organic: amaranth

Arrowhead Mills: organic whole millet

Lundberg Family Farms: organic short-grain brown rice

Lundberg Family Farms: organic brown rice pasta

DeBoles: organic whole-wheat pasta

Ancient Harvest: organic quinoa supergrain pasta

Eddie's Spaghetti: organic vegetable pasta

Pastariso: organic brown rice fettuccine

Pastariso: organic brown rice elbow macaroni

Rising Moon Organics: spinach Florentine ravioli with tofu (F)

Chef Nikola's Kitchen: roasted eggplant in herbed balsamic sauce (F)

Amy's Organic: Asian noodle stir-fry (F)

Amy's Organic: Thai stir-fry (F)

Amy's: roasted vegetable pizza (no cheese) (F)

Nate's: meatless meatballs (F)

Gardein: all products (F)

Health is Wealth: buffalo wings (F)

Health is Wealth: chicken-free patties (F)

Health is Wealth: chicken-free nuggets (F)

Tofurkey: Tofurkey dinner (F)

Gloria's Kitchen: assorted vegan prepared entrees (F)

Lightlife: organic tempeh (R)

Lightlife: Smart Ground (ground "meat") (F)

Nasoya: organic tofu (R)

White Wave: chicken-style seitan (R)

Lightlife: Smart Dogs (R)

Yves: veggie dogs (R)

Rudi's Organic Bakery: white hot dog rolls

Now & Zen: UnChicken (R)

Now & Zen: UnSteak (R)

Yves: Veggie Ground Round Mexican (Mexican-style ground "meat") (F)

Bearitos: taco shells

Garden of Eatin': blue corn taco shells

Alvarado St. Bakery: organic sprouted wheat tortillas

organic vegetables

Obviously, the foods on the lunch and dinner lists can be used interchangeably.

A helpful hint: Prepare large batches of staple food items on Sunday night, to tide you over for your busy workweek. Brown rice, lentils, homemade hummus, soups, and pastas are all good candidates. But try not to do this with your veggies because they'll lose some of their enzymatic punch.

Acceptable Junk Food, Snacks & Desserts

There's something about a snack that makes you feel like a kid again. And that's a good thing. If you're hungry, but not quite ready for dinner, have a small snack. As long as it's healthy, it doesn't spoil your dinner, and if you only have a small serving, there is no reason to feel bad about having a snickety-snack. But don't have one just because you can. Only eat it if you want it. Otherwise, just wait for dinner.

Dessert is one of God's many gifts to humans. Indulge. Like snacks, if your desserts are healthy and eaten in controlled portions, enjoy them without the guilt!

Dr. Cow (www.dr-cow.com): Tree Nut Cheese

Kookie Karma: all products

Sunflour Baking Company: all products

365: organic chocolate soymilk

Whole Foods: organic date coconut rolls

Food Should Taste Good: chips

Nana's Cookie Company: all products

Barbara's Bakery: organic graham crackers

Dagoba: organic dark chocolate bars

Uncle Eddie's: vegan cookies

Organica Foods: vegan cookies

Fabe's All Natural Bakery: vegan cookies, pies, cakes, and macaroons

Laura's Wholesome Junk Food: Bitelettes (cookies)

Soup's On

Nutrilicious Natural Bakery: donut holes

MI-DEL: vanilla snaps

Country Choice: certified organic sandwich cremes

Back to Nature: classic creme sandwich cookies

Back to Nature: chocolate & mint creme sandwich cookies

Chocolove: Belgian dark chocolate

Endangered Species: dark chocolate bars

Tropical Source: rice crisp dark chocolate

Ecco Bella: Health By Chocolate

Raw Balance: Carobelles (www.rawbalance.com) (R)

Gertrude & Bronner's Magic: Alpsnack

LäraBar: all flavors

Terra: exotic vegetable chips original

Terra: spiced sweet potato chips

Maine Coast Sea Vegetables: sea chips

Garden of Eatin': Sunny Blues (tortilla chips with sunflower seeds)

Guiltless Gourmet: yellow corn baked chips

Kettle Organic Tortilla Chips: sesame blue moons

Veggie Stix: shoestring potato sticks

Robert's American Gourmet: Tings

Robert's American Gourmet: Spicy Tings

Robert's American Gourmet: Veggie Booty

Newman's Own: organic salted round pretzels

Koyo Organic Rice Cakes: dulse

Koyo Organic Rice Cakes: mixed grain

Nature's Path: tamari flax crackers

Back to Nature: classic rounds

Soy Dream: non-dairy frozen desserts (F)

Soy Delicious: non-dairy frozen desserts (F)

Soy Delicious: Li'l Buddies ("ice cream" sandwiches) (F)

Purely Decadent: non-dairy frozen dessert (F)

Purely Decadent: coconut milk non-dairy frozen dessert (F)

Azna Gluten-Free: cinnamon rolls, scones (aznaglutenfree.com) (F)

Organic fruit, organic vegetables, organic nuts & seeds

Condiments, Baking Supplies & Miscellaneous

Don't worry about the little odds and ends. We've thought of everything.

Parma: Vegan Parmesan

Earth Balance: natural buttery spread (R)

Soup's On

Soy Garden: natural buttery spread (R)

Follow Your Heart: Vegenaise (mayonnaise substitute) (R)

Nasoya: Nayonaise

Muir Glen: organic ketchup

Westbrae: natural ketchup

Whole Kids: organic yellow mustard

Spectrum Naturals: organic sesame oil

Spectrum Naturals: organic canola oil

Spectrum Naturals: organic extra-virgin olive oil

MaraNatha: organic raw tahini

Bragg Liquid Aminos: all purpose seasoning (soy sauce substitute)

Sea Seasonings: organic kelp granules with cayenne

Annie's Naturals: goddess dressing

OrganicVille: sesame tamari organic vinaigrette

The Wizard's: organic original vegetarian Worcestershire sauce

Essential Living Foods: organic agave nectar or syrup

Shady Maple Farms: certified organic pure maple syrup

Sugar in the Raw: Turbinado sugar from natural cane

Florida Crystals: organic cane sugar

Wholesome Sweeteners: organic sucanat

Hain Pure Foods: organic brown sugar

Stevita Company Inc.: stevia spoonable

Dr. Oetker Organics: chocolate cake mix

Dr. Oetker Organics: vanilla cake mix

Dr. Oetker Organics: chocolate icing mix

Dr. Oetker Organics: vanilla icing mix

Dr. Oetker Organics: chocolate chip cookie mix

Ener-G: egg replacer

Chatfield's Carob & Compliments: dairy-free carob morsels

Sunspire: grain-sweetened chocolate chips

Arrowhead Mills: organic oat flour

Arrowhead Mills: organic whole wheat flour

Arrowhead Mills: organic spelt flour

Arrowhead Mills: organic brown rice flour

Arrowhead Mills: organic blue corn meal

Arrowhead Mills: organic yellow corn meal

Arrowhead Mills: organic flax seeds

Udo's: DHA oil blend

When crafting your own day of eating from the food lists provided, use your head. Create a well-balanced menu for the day without being repetitive. For example, don't eat pancakes for breakfast, a sandwich for lunch, and a veggie burger for dinner. That would be eating all bread, but no fruits or veggies. Duh. Use your head. Try to always think in terms of fruits, veggies, whole grains, and legumes for a well-balanced day of eating.

If you need a little more guidance, feast your eyes on this, a month's worth of menu ideas:

WEEK ONE

Monday

Breakfast: Blueberry pancakes, a banana, soy sausage, and calcium fortified OJ

Lunch: Black bean and lentil burger with lettuce, tomato, and avocado on a whole-grain bun with potato salad

Dinner: Vegetable and tofu curry with rice

Tuesday

Breakfast: Whole-wheat bagel with peanut butter, soy bacon, and a fruit smoothie

Lunch: Grilled tempeh and sauerkraut on a whole-grain bun (with soy mayo and ketchup), served with a salad

Dinner: Fake Chicken patty, baked seasoned potatoes, steamed asparagus

Wednesday

Breakfast: Vegan "Huevos" rancheros made with scrambled tofu, onions, peppers, black beans, avocado and salsa on a whole wheat tortilla

Lunch: Lentil soup and a veggie burger with lettuce and tomato

Dinner: Penne with butternut squash and steamed kale

Thursday

Breakfast: Granola with soy or rice milk with blueberries and strawberries, soy sausage patties, and a grapefruit

Lunch: Burrito with brown rice, black beans, kidney beans, avocado, tomato, and soy cheese

Dinner: Baked ziti with mixed-green salad and garlic bread

Friday

Breakfast: Raisin bran cereal with soy or rice milk, mixed berries and pomegranate juice

Lunch: Veggie Burger with sautéed mushrooms and onions with a side of potato salad

Dinner: Linguini with fake chicken strips, pesto sauce, pine nuts, tomatoes, and faux feta with whole-grain French bread

Soup's On

Saturday

Breakfast: Banana pancakes, tempeh bacon, calcium-fortified OJ

Lunch: Nachos with veggie chili, soy cheese, guacamole, tomatoes and corn chips

Dinner: Spaghetti and soy meatballs with a side salad

Sunday

Breakfast: Oatmeal, raspberry soy yogurt with chopped almonds and grapefruit juice

Lunch: Chilled soba noodles with tofu, snow peas, and red peppers in a sesame peanut sauce

Dinner: Tempeh three bean chili with corn, carrots, and kale and corn muffins

WEEK TWO

Monday

Breakfast: French toast, soy sausage, and a fruit smoothie

Lunch: Minestrone soup, spinach salad, and a multigrain roll

Dinner: Tempeh fajitas with sautéed red and yellow peppers, soy cheese and onions with warm pita bread

Tuesday

Breakfast: English muffin with soy butter and jam, fruit salad and calcium-fortified OJ

Lunch: Vegan sloppy joe's on a whole-grain sesame seed bun with a side of coleslaw

Dinner: Brown rice, broccoli and lentil-stuffed red peppers with a spinach salad

Wednesday

Breakfast: Raisin bran with soy or rice milk, mixed berries, soy sausage, and pomegranate juice

Lunch: Veggie burger with sautéed mushrooms, avocado, lettuce, tomatoes, and onion on a whole-grain roll with roasted sweet potato fries

Dinner: Quesadilla with grilled vegetables, soy cheese, refried beans, avocado, and cilantro

Thursday

Breakfast: Oatmeal, a banana, and a fruit smoothie

Lunch: Club sandwich with fake bacon, faux turkey, soy cheese, lettuce, tomato, and a side of potato salad

Dinner: Teriyaki tofu and veggies over brown rice

Soup's On

Friday

Breakfast: Breakfast burrito with tofu, pinto beans, tomatoes, and rice and a side of fruit

Lunch: Minestrone soup, with a hummus and veggie wrap

Dinner: Brown rice with a fake chicken patty and sautéed kale, broccoli, and garlic

Saturday

Breakfast: Blueberry pancakes with tempeh bacon and calcium-fortified OJ

Lunch: Sub sandwich with baked eggplant slices, mushrooms, and pizza sauce on a multi-grain sub roll and a side salad

Dinner: Nachos with chili, soy cheese, guacamole, scallions, tomatoes and corn chips

Sunday

Breakfast: Tempeh sausage with biscuits and gravy, fruit salad, and grapefruit juice

Lunch: Take-out veggie sushi, miso soup, side salad, and a spring roll

Dinner: Baked stuffed shells with tomato sauce, a side salad, and garlic bread

WEEK THREE

Monday

Breakfast: Toaster waffles with bananas and strawberries, soy yogurt, and calcium-fortified OJ

Lunch: Club sandwich with fake bacon, faux turkey, avocado, lettuce, and mayo with a chickpea side salad

Dinner: Veggie pizza with a Caesar salad

Tuesday

Breakfast: Oatmeal, half a cantaloupe, and grapefruit juice

Lunch: Pita wrap with grilled zucchini, mushrooms, eggplant, and hummus, with a handful of grapes

Dinner: Vegetable potpie with a mixed green salad and bread

Wednesday

Breakfast: Blueberry muffin with soy cream cheese and tempeh bacon, fruit salad, and decaf green tea

Lunch: Lentil and bean burger with soy cheese, avocado, and tomato on a whole-grain bun with a side of oven-baked seasoned fries

Dinner: Whole-wheat spaghetti with fake meatballs, tomato sauce, mixed-green salad, and garlic bread

Soup's On

Thursday

Breakfast: Tofu scramble with mushrooms, red peppers and garlic, with toast and jam and a fruit smoothie

Lunch: Leftover spaghetti and soy meatballs

Dinner: Shepherd's pie with mashed potatoes, lentils, carrots, and peas with a side salad

Friday

Breakfast: Granola with strawberries, fake bacon, and orange juice

Lunch: Vegetable and bean burrito with avocado and salsa

Dinner: Veggie lasagna with eggplant, zucchini, red peppers, small mixed green salad, and whole-grain garlic bread

Saturday

Breakfast: Waffles, cantaloupe, and apple juice

Lunch: Grilled portobello mushroom sandwich with red pepper pesto, lettuce, tomatoes, and soy cheese on a whole-grain bun with a bowl of broccoli soup

Dinner: Thai tofu stir-fry with bok choy, snow peas, and whole-wheat soba noodles

Sunday

Breakfast: Bagel with peanut butter, a side of soy sausage, and almond milk

Lunch: Vegetable fajitas with a side of beans and rice

Dinner: Homemade pizza with vegetables, soy cheese, and soy pepperoni

WEEK FOUR

Monday

Breakfast: Cereal with almond milk, fruit salad, and calcium-fortified OJ

Lunch: Veggie burger with sautéed onions, mushrooms, and peppers, and a side of potato salad

Dinner: Spaghetti with fake meatballs and tomato sauce, a mixed green salad, and garlic bread

Tuesday

Breakfast: Fried tofu sandwich with soy cheese and soy bacon on a whole-wheat bagel and pomegranate juice

Lunch: Grilled zucchini and portabella mushroom wrap with a side of oven-baked fries

Dinner: Vegetable paella with soy chorizo

Wednesday

Breakfast: Peppers, onions, and veggie sausage in a whole-wheat tortilla, calcium-fortified OJ

Lunch: Veggie chili with carrots, avocado, tomato, and cilantro and an apple

Dinner: BBQ tofu "ribs" with garlic mashed potatoes and corn on the cob

Thursday

Breakfast: French toast with strawberries and raspberries and fresh-squeezed apple juice

Lunch: Lentil burger with sautéed mushrooms, and lettuce, tomato on a whole-grain bun with coleslaw

Dinner: Tacos with soy meat crumbles, soy cheese, black beans, guacamole, and salsa

Friday

Breakfast: Oatmeal with raisins, berries, and banana and an orange juice

Lunch: Chilled soba noodles with tofu, snow peas, and broccoli in a sesame peanut sauce

Dinner: Burrito with pinto beans, brown rice, soy cheese, guacamole, and tomatoes

Saturday

Breakfast: Tofu scramble with veggies and roasted potatoes, fruit smoothie

Lunch: Caesar salad with fake chicken strips and croutons and a whole-grain roll

Dinner: Baked teriyaki tempeh with brown rice and steamed green beans

Sunday

Breakfast: Pancakes with soy sausage and a fruit salad

Lunch: Macaroni and soy cheese and a side salad

Dinner: Vegetable curry

*Feel free to snack on a handful of raw organic nuts each day. And if you really want to treat yourself right, have fresh-squeezed veggie juice every day. (Fresh-squeezed, not packaged or pasteurized.)

**Don't forget to drink eight glasses of water a day.

***We include a list of recommended cookbooks toward the end of the book. Buy a book or use the Internet for easy vegan recipes. One great site, veganpeace.com, includes recipes and a review of veggie cookbooks.

Chapter 13

FYI

Um, just 'cause we wrote this book doesn't mean we're perfect. We like to pig out, loaf around, and tie one on from time to time. So if you see us eating junk food or doing beer bongs, don't hold it against us—we're human. For the most part, we take good care of ourselves, so when we do treat our bodies like shit, we don't feel the least bit bad about it.

൭

Yeah, eating onions and garlic makes your breath smell like someone took a shit down your throat. But they fight cancer and help detoxify your liver. So eat 'em.

൭

What's all the drama surrounding hydrogenated oils? Manufacturers add hydrogen to mono- or polyunsaturated fats (good fats) to change their consistency. The end result, trans-fatty acid (bad), is a more solid product with a longer shelf life. Margarines, cookies, cakes, doughnuts, potato chips, meat and dairy products, and shortening can contain hydrogenated oils. Trans-fatty acids can cause derangements of cell structure, accelerated aging, and a predisposition to diseases.[548]

Think about it. They are literally altering a naturally occurring product's molecular structure by adding hydrogen molecules to it. Eating these chemically altered foods containing hydrogenated oils will increase your risk of heart disease. Sadly, heating oil at high temperatures also changes its natural molecular configuration and produces free-radicals. Free-radicals not only destroy essential fats and vitamins but also are linked with cancer and heart disease.[549] This is why olive or peanut oils, which are healthy, can be very *unhealthy* in dishes like fried eggplant or French fries. Avoid eating fried foods (sniffle) and reusing heated oils. Never heat oil to the point where it is smoking. Cook with canola or coconut oil using low heat and for the shortest amount of time possible.

ଔ

Don't be a cheap asshole. Yeah, yeah, yeah, organic produce is usually more expensive than conventional produce. But you spend countless dollars on stupid boy stuff, rent or mortgages, car payments, and other bullshit. Surely your health and body are more important than anything else in your life (you only get one body). Even if you are spending more on organic food, you'll save money in the long run by preparing more meals and snacks at home—always cheaper than buying food on the fly. If you can afford it, organic is worth the extra money, and you should aim to have everything you eat be organic, but especially fruits or vegetables that you eat without peeling the skin. Always buy organic blueberries, strawberries, raspberries, apples, and pears. Peanuts and peanut butter, too, because conventional ones are loaded with pesticides. Buying organic produce is the only way to guarantee you're not eating genetically modified organisms. According to *Food Additives: A Shopper's Guide to What's Safe & What's Not*, "genes are taken from one species of plant, animal, or virus and inserted into another species in order to produce a desirable trait, such as disease resistance or hardier crops. No one knows the long-term effects of eating genetically modified foods. Genetically modified foods are being sold now and they are not being labeled. Certified organic foods are the only foods guaranteed not to be genetically modified."[550] So do the best you can and buy organic food whenever it's available. (But don't be a neurotic freak when it's not available.)

⁓

Two or three times a day, every day for your entire life, you swallow trace amounts of toothpaste. What's in it? Chemicals? Artificial sweeteners? Would you eat it? Read the ingredients. Buy natural.

⁓

The skin is the body's largest organ. Every day, we slop all sorts of potions and lotions on ourselves and rub them into our skin. Ever read the ingredients of these products? Ever consider that you are putting chemicals directly onto your largest organ? Ever think about the pores all over your body and what you're putting inside them? Hopefully, you will now. Buy natural products. What you put on your body is just as important as what you put in your body (because, in essence, what you put *on* your body will wind up *in* your body), especially on body parts you shave. Open pores do not want chemicals bulldozing through. Are your deodorant, shaving cream, cologne, and lotions safe?

⁓

Natural, unrefined Celtic sea salt (different from table salt) contains many essential minerals, enhances organ function, and neutralizes toxins. It also contributes to the hydration of our cells and organs.[551]

⁓

FYI

Buy a food steamer. It will change your life.

附

Do yoga. Not only are you guaranteed to meet hot yoga bunnies, but it is also a kick-ass cardio workout that will strengthen, tone, and harden your muscles. Yoga is amazing for organ function, immune system strength, tackling insomnia, and improving overall health. You will love how it makes you look and feel. (Yes, real men do yoga.) All kidding aside, if everyone did yoga, we would have world peace.

附

Donate blood. You can save a life and lose weight at the same time.

附

Keep your eyes peeled for bad press regarding veganism. It's usually planted by the industries that are threatened by the movement. Don't believe any of it. It's all bogus bullshit. One study claimed that feeding children a vegan diet was tantamount to child abuse. It just so happens that the National Cattlemen's Beef Association paid for the study. They had the gall to experiment on African children who were literally starving. These children were eating nothing but corn and beans in minuscule servings. When servings of meat were added to their diets, their health improved.[552] Well, of course it did. They were fucking starving. This doesn't prove that veganism is dangerous or unhealthy. It just shows that the National Cattlemen's Beef Association will exploit starving, impoverished children to create bad press for veganism and boost its own meat sales. This is nothing short of a disgrace and an embarrassment to America.

Chapter 14

Use Your (Big) Head

Don't be a fat slob anymore. You know what you have to do, now do it. But don't go manorexic on us, either. It's easy to get caught up in any lifestyle change and go overboard. Make healthy choices and take excellent care of yourself without getting neurotic and obsessive.

USE YOUR HEAD. We can't say it enough. Use your own head and think about what you are eating. Forget what you've ever read, heard, or learned and just think for yourself. Once they've recovered, your body, brain, and instincts will always lead you down the right food path. Obey them and disregard everyone and everything else. You know the truth.

Read the ingredients. This goes hand in hand with using your head. If you plan on eating something, you should know exactly what it is. Even if it's a product that we've recommended, you still need to check the ingredients. Companies change their recipes all the time. Two vegan products we loved and suggested weren't vegan by the time we were finished writing this book, and we had to remove them from our recommendation lists. Trust no one. Not even us. Some of the products on our suggested food lists aren't perfect; we make certain allowances based on our own opinions and desires. Read and decide for yourself. And if you don't recognize an ingredient, call the company's toll-free number on the package and ask what it is. If it's not something you would put in your body, tell them, and suggest that they improve their product. Companies really do take comments into account, so always voice your opinion.

Now that you're a *Skinny Bastard*, don't turn into a skinny bastard. We conceived the titles of our books *Skinny Bitch* and *Skinny Bastard* to get attention. We just wanted to spread our message far and wide and thought this was a good way to do it. But we are not bitches, we hate men who are bastards, and we have no desire to promote douchey behavior. There is nothing uglier than a hot guy who's an asshole. If you look great, you should feel good about yourself and be happy. Instead of fixating on the last five pounds you want to lose, celebrate the five you already lost. Progress, not perfection. While

Use Your (Big) Head

women aren't hung up on landing a guy who's gorgeous, we are hung up on guys who are sweet, funny, and confident. Don't be insecure or competitive or feel threatened by guys who are richer or hotter or who have more hair than you. Respect them; it will make you look better.

Soon, you'll notice people (especially women, but some gay guys, too) flocking to the new you. Not just because you're buff but because you are happier, healthier, and eating a cruelty-free diet. So feel free to share your new wealth of information with everyone who asks. Spread the good word, but be careful not to preach. You'll see that some people get very defensive about their diets when you tell them about yours. Even if you are being nonjudgmental, people may feel threatened by your stance. Understandably, your being vegan shines a spotlight on the cruelty they're contributing to, and it makes them feel uncomfortable. When asked, you can describe what you've learned about the treatment of farm animals and all of the health benefits of being vegan. By all means, let people know how great you feel and how much weight you've lost. But never suggest that they try it or make them feel bad about their diet. Offer to lend them your copy of *Skinny Bastard* or give them the GoVeg.com website. But don't cram it down their throats. Everyone seeks the truth in his or her own time.

Now that you've got your diet, health, and appearance under control, fix other areas of your life. After all, there's no point in being shredded if your life is a mess. Repair or end your co-dependent relationship, quit your dead-end job, and ditch your lame-ass friends. Make a list of goals and start chipping away at them. THIS IS YOUR LIFE! Live it to the fullest with reckless abandon. Seize the day. And do it again tomorrow. Live. Go get your dream job. Search for your dream girl (or guy). Fear nothing. Try everything. Be excited. You'll never get yesterday back, but today is yours for the taking. Make it great.

Bravo. You've got your life and your diet on track. But you still need to move your ass. Exercise will boost your self-esteem, reduce your junk-food cravings, and help you *lose weight*. Being physically fit can also reduce your risk of stroke by up to 40 percent![553] (Stroke is our nation's third leading cause of death.)[554] If you can commit to a gym routine, fantastic! You will reach your fitness goals faster. But you don't need to be a gym rat. Just do something! It can even be fun. Take a kickboxing class or go to a "bootcamp." Go for walks after dinner or bike rides on weekends. Better yet, walk or bike to work or the commuter train. Whatever you choose, exercise makes you feel great about yourself. And that alone is priceless.

Use Your (Big) Head

You *are* what you *think*. Our thoughts, feelings, beliefs, and experiences create tangible, concrete reactions at cellular and atomic levels. So whether something is "real" or not doesn't matter. If we think, feel, believe, or experience it, it will become a reality. Slow down and think about this and realize the implications it can have on your life. It can work for or against you. For example, if you *think* you are fat and that diets never work and that you'll always be fat, then yes, you are fat and diets never work and you will always be fat. What you *think* actually becomes embedded in your brain and your cells and the energy field surrounding you. Your thoughts are that powerful. So if you *feel* you are meant to be lean and *believe* this lifestyle will make you lose weight and *know* that this book is going to change your life, you *will* be lean, you *will* lose weight, and your life *will* change. It is just that simple.

In her book, *Anatomy of the Spirit*, Dr. Caroline Myss examines the unquestionable link between negative emotions and physical illnesses. Take "Julie," for example. Julie's husband treated her with contempt and disdain, frequently said the mere sight of her repulsed him, and refused to sleep with her. It is no coincidence that Julie was diagnosed with breast and ovarian cancer, reflecting her lack of self-love for her "womanhood." She could not leave her husband, never recovered from her cancer, and died as a result.[555] "Joanna" was married to a man who had multiple affairs that she knew about but tried to live with. Not surprisingly, she developed breast cancer. Eventually, she confronted her husband and demanded fidelity. However, he was unable to change, so she left the marriage. Joanna recovered from her cancer.[556] *Anatomy of the Spirit* chronicles one history after another of people sickening themselves or healing themselves with thought and emotion. (Of course, we are not suggesting that everyone suffering from a disease has brought it upon him- or herself. We are, however, saying it is entirely possible to do so.)

Our minds are infinitely powerful. Our favorite self-help gurus, Dr. Wayne Dyer, Louise Hay, and Anthony (Tony) Robbins, understand this, and they all preach the power of daily affirmations. An affirmation is a positive statement you make that allows you to clearly envision an achieved goal or mindset. It is declared as if it is already happening, and it can be anything you want:

"Every day in every way I'm losing more and more weight."

"Every day in every way my body is getting leaner."

"Every day in every way my stomach is getting flatter."

"Every day in every way my muscles are getting bigger."

Use Your (Big) Head

"Every day in every way I'm loving my body more."

"Every day in every way I'm getting healthier and healthier."

Create your own affirmations and say them (in your head or aloud, if you can) when you wake up in the morning, while exercising, in your car, and in bed at night. You will immediately notice how good they make you feel and be astonished at the results. This book is the result of our affirmations, so we *know* they truly work.

You worked hard for this body, and you shouldn't waste it by covering it up in crappy clothes. So take your ass on a shopping spree and upgrade your wardrobe. We know it can feel a little strange, paying so much attention to your looks—like you don't have the right or aren't worthy. But you *are* good enough, you *do* deserve it, and no one is thinking otherwise. This is your body for this lifetime. Dress it well and love it. If you have poor fashion sense (you know who you are), ask someone for guidance.

Now we know we keep encouraging you to look your best, but, for the love of God, don't associate your worth with your appearance. We are spiritual beings walking around in these crazy bodies. Our insides are much more important than our outsides. So don't you dare measure your worth by the amount of attention or validation you get from women. It's nice to be appreciated, but it is not a necessity. Love yourself and your looks, even if no one else seems to. In time, your confidence and self-love will attract a winner.

Well, it's all there in black and white. We sincerely hope you will take the knowledge you've learned and put it to use from this moment on. YOU hold the power to change your life, and it's really so simple. Use your head, lose your ass.

Isn't man an amazing animal? He kills wildlife by the millions in order to protect his domestic animals and their feed. Then he kills domestic animals by the billions and eats them. This in turn kills man by the millions, because eating all those animals leads to degenerative—and fatal—health conditions like heart disease, kidney disease, and cancer. So then man tortures and kills millions more animals to look for cures for these diseases. Elsewhere, millions of other human beings are being killed by hunger and malnutrition because food they could eat is being used to fatten domestic animals. Meanwhile, some people are dying of sad laughter at the absurdity of man, who kills so easily and so violently, and once a year sends out cards praying for "Peace on Earth."[557]

—*Old MacDonald's Factory Farm*, by C. David Coates

New Afterwords by the Authors

Rory Freedman

Instead of calling our first book *Skinny Bitch*, it could just as easily have been titled *Sneaky Bitch*.

After years of radio, television, and print interviews, you get kinda sick of hearing yourself say the same things over and over again. But there's one topic I never get tired of discussing, however, ironically, it's one I often shy away from when I'm doing mainstream interviews.

While the book has been successful—translations in more than twenty languages, millions of copies in print, two years on the *New York Times* Best Seller list—there has been one constant criticism: Nowhere on the cover or back cover does is it reveal that we're promoting a vegan diet.

Well, the jig is up—I'm coming clean. My primary motivation for writing the *Skinny Bitch* series was to educate people about factory farming and slaughterhouses. Sixteen years ago, I had been eating meat at every meal. But the day I read a magazine article about how animals are confined, brutalized, and killed—all because we like how their flesh tastes—that was it for me. I called myself an animal lover; how could I contribute to that?

We are a society of animal lovers. And when I had the idea for the book, I firmly believed, just as I do now, that when people learn about factory farming and slaughterhouses, they, too, will be horrified and compelled enough to change their diets. The only problem was, and is: No one wants to sit down and read a book that talks about these horrors. That's when it occurred to me: If there were a book about the subject, it was called *Skinny Bitch*, and it didn't advertise its content, people would read it and get the message.

The rest is history. I called Kim that same day and told her my idea. She had already been bugging me to go into some sort of health-related business with her, so she was onboard immediately. For months, we had been talking about how tragic it was that people were dying of cancer left and right and that animals were being killed—and that those two things were totally linked. We both desperately wanted to change the world but didn't quite know how. *Skinny Bitch* was the vehicle we were looking for.

But if you see, read, or hear one of my interviews, it's possible I'll be downplaying the vegan aspect of the book. While I want nothing more than to talk about the issue, I know that in the short time or space I'm allotted, I'm not going to make a compelling enough argument for veganism. But if I discuss the parts of *Skinny Bitch* or *Skinny Bastard* that people can more easily relate to, and then they get the book, I know they'll be getting a well-crafted, well researched, comprehensive argument about veganism.

The "v" word seems to be better known now than ever before in history. With ever-increasing awareness about animal cruelty, environmental issues, and meat- and dairy-related diseases and health problems, more and more people are getting on the veg train. That said, veganism is still as loathsome to some people as ever before. Why? Where does this hatred come from? A recent study in *Psychology Today* explained this unfortunate phenomenon. Basically, the ego is so strong that in order to protect oneself from thinking, "I'm a bad person," it instead offers, "you're a bad person." It's a bitter pill to swallow that you're contributing to animals being skinned alive, just because you like meat. It's much easier to think that vegetarians are pains in the asses, have no lives, and are hippie-crunchy losers. Granted, many vegetarians are annoying, have no lives, and are hippie-crunchy losers. But most of us are normal people; we just don't want animals harmed.

So why now? Why am I showing my cards now, after all this time? I just finished reading *Power vs. Force* by David Hawkins, and one of the things he talks about is how the human body can detect truth and righteousness, even when the mind cannot. I realized that no matter what, if I spoke the truth, it would be the right thing.

So here it is. The truth is that animals are innocent beings, and there is no justification for the brutality inflicted upon them. And I was put on this earth to try and educate others about what happens on farms and in slaughterhouses—to motivate people to stop eating animals. The truth is that in the United States alone, ten billion land animals are killed every year for human consumption. And no matter what you say about the food chain, or how you were raised, or how you "could never give up meat," you cannot begin to imagine the sheer horror of what you're contributing to every time you sit down to eat.

Since our first book came out in 2005, I've often heard myself saying during interviews, "This book is not for everyone." And it's true—it's not for everyone. Some people will read *Skinny Bitch* or *Skinny Bastard* and be totally furious that they promote a vegan diet.

And while they contain a ton of other compelling, life-changing information, they just won't be able to get past the veganism. These books are not for everyone. They're for people who want to be healthy. They're for people who want to eat well. They're for people who love food. They're for people who have tried everything else. But most of all, they are for people who want to live in the truth. People who are tired of being lied to and who are tired of lying to themselves. People who know they can do better and who want to do better. People who want to take that long, hard look in the mirror and ask, "What am I responsible for here?"

While educating people about animals was my primary motivation for writing *Skinny Bitch*, I also wanted to help humans. So many people are suffering from weight problems, disease, and depression, and diet is almost always the reason. But so many people just can't grasp that. They just aren't ready, willing, or able to let go of their excuses, none of which serve them at all. My ultimate goal in writing *Skinny Bitch* (and the four other books that followed) then, which is the same now, was that people would get inspired by and excited about the idea of change. That they would get so revved up reading the book that

New Afterwords by the Authors

maybe, for the first time ever, change would be exhilarating and invigorating and not overwhelming and daunting. Based on the thousands of e-mails we've received from all over the world, I know people are absolutely rising to the challenge, and nothing could be more beautiful.

This book is not for everyone. It's for you.

—Rory, 2009

Kim Barnouin

The past few years, since our first book *Skinny Bitch* came out, have been amazing. If I take a step back and think about the incredible journey that the *Skinny Bitch* series has taken me on, I'm still in awe. The vast majority of people I meet have either read or heard of the books. I think the moment it hit me that we had really done something big was when I started to read the thousands of e-mails from fans all over the world—from every age group, gender, and ethnicity—who shared inspirational success stories: how their lives were improved after changing their diet, how much weight they lost and how they were able to play with their children again as a result, how their allergies and skin cleared up, how their cholesterol levels dropped, how they became interested in studying nutrition to pass on the message of healthy eating, how new animal advocates got inspired to make a difference. All these stories and more were because of something I was a part of. And to all the people who shared their stories with us, thank you so much; you have touched me too.

I remember the beginning of this journey with Rory. I'd been harassing her relentlessly to go into business with me to promote health and wellness—but I had no idea what that meant for us. All I knew was that I had been suffering from some health issues, and through lots of research I discovered the healing power of nutrition. I changed my diet, dumped a majority of the unhealthy foods (and the list was long!), and noticed how my body reacted to healthy foods. I healed myself mentally and physically, which led to starting my Master's degree in nutrition, with the goal of helping others heal themselves with food. Through the course of my studies, I was shocked to learn about all the illnesses and diseases in our country and how nutrition plays a significant role in the development and healing of many of them.

Finally Rory called me and said, "Okay, let's do something. I know how to start this: We are going to write a book." Once we decided to write the book, it was as if the planets aligned just for us. We got referred to an amazing literary agent, who has always been our rock. We laugh now at how so many publishing companies turned us down in 2004, many of whom weren't ready to publish and promote a book titled *Skinny Bitch*. But lucky for us, our phenomenal publishing company Running Press believed in our vision, and has continued to do so five books later.

Skinny **Bastard**

And the journey has taken us far! We have passed the 100-week mark on the *New York Times* Best Seller list for *Skinny Bitch*. We've sold millions of books. And we've touched the lives of hundreds of thousands of people—families who are living better because of us.

I initially wondered how readers would respond to the topics in *Skinny Bitch* (and in the male counterpart, *Skinny Bastard*). Would they be open to giving up diet soda and dairy if they knew the dark sides of these foods? Would they want to hear about the treatment of factory farm animals, or would they cover their ears, thinking what they don't know won't hurt them? Throughout the book, we talked about poop, we bitched about the USDA, and we asked a lot of questions about what was going into our food. We wrapped it with a clever title, peppered it with laugh-out-loud funny bits, and included lots of hard research to back up our claims. It certainly wasn't a new diet made up by Rory and me, but it was a little off the beaten path. I am still amazed that so many people from all over the world have at best embraced a new way of eating and at least have a better understanding of health and nutrition and the important role it plays in our life.

I love it when people come up to me and tell me that our books convinced them to give up an unhealthy food or add a healthy food and go on to report how it specifically changed their health. I met a woman at an event recently who said she no longer drinks diet soda because a friend of hers read that chapter and called her immediately to tell her to stop drinking it. And now both women know exactly why it's not a healthy drink. People are listening! I constantly hear how upon giving up dairy the weight flew off, especially those last five pounds. I can see their glowing skin as proof of their success. Others tell me that they can go grocery shopping much better prepared now— they know what ingredients to stay away from and why, and they choose healthier alternatives. I am proud when I hear people talking about what's in our food and question why it's there. That's been my goal all along: to guide people on making healthier choices. I wanted to get people asking questions and researching for themselves what they were putting into their bodies. I wanted people to read our books and be inspired to make some changes in their diet. Big or small, it doesn't matter—everything in life is a process, and I certainly didn't get there overnight. It took me years to change my diet, and I am still not perfect. I'm definitely a junk-food lover at heart, but by building a healthy foundation daily, I can still enjoy my treats and not feel bad.

People often ask me how to get their family involved in healthier eating. Here's what I did: I bought as many cookbooks as I could afford (as well as co-writing our own, *Skinny Bitch in the Kitch*) and declared that I would be cooking on most nights. I would make dinner, put everything on the table, and not discuss details about the ingredients—just simply let my family eat. My cooking has certainly gotten better—and I've become very creative in the process. Not only is food supposed to be enjoyable, preparing it should be as well! Be open to trying the new ingredients introduced in this book—and remember just because it's new doesn't mean it's not fun, tasty, and satisfying. As I follow my path in nutrition and wellness, I will continue to learn, to educate, and hopefully inspire people to enjoy food in a healthy way. I hope you enjoy our *Skinny Bitch* books as much as I do, and that they change the way you look at food.

—Kim, 2009

Recommended Reading

Books

Slaughterhouse, Gail A. Eisnitz.
*This book is an absolute must-read for every American who has ever eaten meat, is still considering eating meat, or isn't sure if they should or shouldn't. Buy this book today!

Breaking the Food Seduction, Neal Barnard, M.D.

Carbophobia: The Sorry Truth About America's Low-Carb Craze, Michael Greger, M.D.

The China Study,
T. Colin Campbell, Ph.D. and Tomas M. Campbell, II

Diet For a Poisoned Planet, David Steinman

Dominion, Matthew Scully

Eat More, Weigh Less, Dean Ornish, M.D.

Fast Food Nation, Eric Schlosser

The Food Revolution, John Robbins

The McDougall Program,
John McDougall, M.D. and Mary McDougall

Prevent and Reverse Heart Disease, Caldwell B. Esselstyn, Jr., M.D.

The Way We Eat, Jim Mason and Peter Singer

Cookbooks

Skinny Bitch in the Kitch,
yours truly, Rory Freedman and Kim Barnouin

The Uncheese Cookbook, Joanne Stepaniak

The Garden of Vegan, Tanya Barnard and Sara Kramer

How it All Vegan, by Tanya Barnard and Sara Kramer

The Compassionate Cook, PETA and Ingrid Newkirk

CalciYum, David and Rachelle Bronfman

The Native Foods Restaurant Cookbook, Tanya Petrovna

The Candle Café Cookbook,
Joy Pierson and Bart Potenza with Barbara Scott-Goodman

Vegan Planet, Robin Robertson

Veganomicon,
Isa Chandra Moskowitz and Terry Hope Romero

Viva le Vegan!, Dreena Burton

Very Vegetarian, Jannequin Bennet

The Vegan Table,
Colleen Patrick Goudreau

The Joy of Vegan Baking,
Colleen Patrick Goudreau

Veganpeace.com offers recipes and reviews of veggie cookbooks

Restaurant Guides

happycow.net

(This site is heaven on Earth! You can find all the veggie-friendly restaurants in your 'hood, and, when you travel, you can make sure you know all the local haunts.)

vegoutguide.com

Websites

goveg.com

pcrm.org

cok.net

VeganOutreach.org

oa.org (overeaters anonymous), 505-891-2664

thediscerningbrute.com

Food Websites

goveg.com

veganstore.com

rawbalance.com

playfood.org

deliciouschoices.com

TreeHugginTreats.com

simpletreats.com

chocolatedecadence.com

leaheyfoods.com

vegandreams.com

goodbaker.com

rosecitychocolates.com

eatraw.com

nutrilicious.com

allisonsgourmet.com

healthy-eating.com

Merchandise Websites

veganstore.com

VeganEssentials.com

AlternativeOutfitters.com

feelgoodtees.com

mooshoes.com

veganunlimited.com

TheVegetarianSite.com

VegSexShop.com

Sources Consulted

Abel, Barbara. "Men and Heart Disease; Take Lifestyle Cues from Women." Medicalcollegeofwisconcin.edu, May 2005; accessed Dec. 5, 2008,
http://healthlink.mcw.edu/article/1031002509.html

Anderson JW. "Dietary fiber in nutrition management of diabetes."
In: G. Vahouny V, and D. Kritchevsky, eds., *Dietary Fiber: Basic and Clinical Aspects,* pp. 343-360. New York: Plenum Press, 1986.

Armstrong, Clare, MS, RD. DiscoveryHealth.com. The Discovery Channel, updated Sept. 25, 2002; accessed Jan. 20, 2005,
http://health.discovery.com/encyclopedias/1940.html

Aronson, Dina, MS, RD. Interviewed by Rory Freedman, May 17, 2007.

Aronson, Dina. "The Soy and Male Fertility Study." Veganrd.com, July 25, 2008; accessed Nov. 24, 2008,
http://www.veganrd.blogspot.com/2008/07/soy-and-male-fertility-study.html

Aspartame Victims Support Group, updated Jan. 13, 2005; accessed Jan. 20, 2005, http://www.presidiotex.com/aspartame/

Associated Press. Study Links Childrens Asthma to Hog Farms. ABC News, December 2004; accessed March 11, 2005,
http://abcnews.go.com/Health/wireStory?id=317383

Atkins, Robert C., MD. *Dr. Atkins' New Diet Revolution.* New York: Avon, 2002.

Baillie-Hamilton, Paula, MD, PhD. *The Body Restoration Plan.* New York: Avery, 2003.

"Bad Breath, Foods and Eating." Kissmegoodnight.com; accessed Dec. 7, 2008, http://www.kissmegoodnight.com/bad-breath/bad-breath-food-eating.shtml

"Banned as Human Food, StarLink Corn Found in Food Aid." *Environmental News Service,* Feb. 16, 2005; accessed Feb. 20, 2005, http://www.ens-newswire.com/ens/feb2005/2005-02-16-09.asp#anchor2

"Barcelona Report," Jan. 12, 2005; accessed Dec. 1, 2008, http://www.presidiotex.com/barcelona/

Barnard, Neal MD. *Breaking the Food Seduction: The Hidden Reasons Behind Food Cravings—and 7 Steps to End Them Naturally.* New York: St. Martins Press, 2003.

Barnard, Neal, MD. "Nutrition and Prostate Health." Thecancerproject.org; accessed Oct. 25, 2008, http://www.cancerproject.org/survival/cancer_facts/prostate_health.php

Barnard, Neal, MD. "Meat Too Tough to Eat." Pcrm.org, published in *Hartford Courant,* accessed Sept. 14, 2007, http://www.pcrm.org/news/082806.html

Barnard, Neal MD. "Milk and Prostate Cancer: The Evidence Mounts." Pcrm.org; accessed Oct. 25, 2008, http://www.pcrm.org/health/prevmed/milk_prostate.html

Barnard, Neal, MD. "Prostate Cancer: Prevention and Survival." Thecancerproject.org; accessed Oct. 25, 2008, http://www.cancerproject.org/survival/cancer_facts/prostate.php

Barnard, Neal, MD. *The Power of Your Plate.* Summertown, TN: Book Publishing Company, 1990, pp. 25-6.

Beck, Leslie, R.D. *The Ultimate Nutrition Guide for Women: How to Stay Healthy with Diet, Vitamins, Minerals, and Herbs.* Hoboken: John Wiley & Sons, 2001.

Sources

Bellon, Roberta. National Justice League. "Aspartame Lawsuits Accuse Many Companies of Poisoning the Public," April 6, 2004, accessed Feb. 10, 2005, http://www.newmediaexplorer.org/sepp/2004/04/09/aspartame_neurotoxic_coca_cola_pepsi_nutra_sweet_sued_in_california.htm

Betts, Debra. "Male Fertility." Rhizone.net; accessed Oct. 25, 2008, http://acupuncture.rhizome.net.nz/infertility-men.aspx

Billy, Thomas J. "FSIS Case Study—Meat and Poultry HACCP," July 13, 1999, accessed Jan. 9, 2009, http://www.fsis.usda.gov/OA/speeches/1999/tb_forum.htm.

"Blood Pressure and Coffee Consumption." Menwell.com, Apr. 2008; accessed Nov. 25, 2008, http://www.menwell.com.au/news/blood-pressure-and-coffee-consumption/

Bookspan, Jolie. MEd, PhD, FAWN. "World Vegan Day Is November 1." Healthline.com, Nov.1, 2007; accessed Nov. 23, 2008, http://www.healthline.com/blogs/exercise_fitness/2007/11/world-vegan-day-is-november-1.html

Boschen, Hank. "Cycles of the Body," Juiceguy.com, Feb. 10, 2005; accessed Dec. 1, 2008, http://www.juiceguy.com/cycle.shtml

Bray, George A., Samara Joy Nielson, and Barry M. Popkin. "Consumption of high-fructose corn syrup in beverages may play a role in the epidemic of obesity." *American Journal of Clinical Nutrition,* vol. 79, no. 4, 537-543, Apr. 2004, http://www.ajcn.org/cgi/content/abstract/79/4/537

Brazier, Brendan. "The High Performance Vegan Athlete: It is Possible." Vegkitchen.com; accessed Dec. 5, 2008, http://vegkitchen.com/tips/vegan-athlete.htm

Brown, Harold. E-mail to Rory Freedman, March 21, 2005.

Brownell, Kelly D., *Food Fight: The Inside Story of the Food Industry, Americas Obesity Crisis & What We Can Do About It.* New York, McGraw Hill: 2004

Brownlee, Christen. *The Beef About UTIs,* Jan. 15, 2005; accessed Jan. 20, 2005, http://www.sciencenews.org/articles/20050115/food.asp

Buhner, Stephen Harrod. *The Natural Testosterone Plan: For Sexual Health and Energy.* Rochester, VT: Healing Arts Press, 2007.

Burros, Marian. "Splendas Sugar Claim Unites Odd Couple of Nutrition Wars." *New York Times*, Feb.15, 2005; accessed Feb. 20, 2005, query.nytimes.com/gst/fullpage.html?res=aCOCEODF123AF936a25751C O49639C8D63

Butler RN, Lewis MI, Hoffman E, Whitehead ED. "Love and sex after 60," *Geriatrics.* 1994;49(10):27-32.

Caffeine. eCureMe Inc., Feb. 10, 2005, http://life.ecureme.com/ healthyliving/naturalmedicine/n_caffeine.asp

"Calcium and Strong Bones." Pcrm.org; accessed Oct. 25, 2008, http://pcrm.org/health/prevmed/strong_bones.html

Campbell, T. Colin, PhD, and Thomas M. Campbell II. *The China Study. Startling Implications for Diet, Weight Loss and Long-Term Health.* Dallas, TX: Benbella Books, 2006.

"Cancer Facts—Colon Cancer." Cancerproject.org; accessed Oct. 25, 2008, http://www.cancerproject.org/survival/cancer_facts/colon.php

"Cancer Facts—Meat Consumption and Cancer Risk." Cancerproject.org; accessed Nov. 25, 2008,

Sources

http://www.cancerproject.org/survival/cancer_facts/meat.php

Caplan, Jeff. "Go-To and Tofu Guy: Stack Makes Switch." *Fort Worth Star Telegram,* Nov. 23, 2007, p. C1.

Caring Consumer Guide. Peta.org, March 26, 2005, http://www.caringconsumer.com/ingredientslist.html

"A Cesspool of Pollutants. Now Is the Time to Clean Up Your Body." Nealhendrickson.com. August, 2004; accessed Mar. 6, 2007, http://www.nealhendrickson.com/mcdougall/2004nl/040800pucesspool.htm

Chan, June M, Meir Jo, Stampfer, Jing, Ma, Peter H Gann, J Michael Gaziano, Edward L Giovannucci. "Dairy products, calcium, and prostate cancer risk in the Physicians' Health Study." *The American Journal of Clinical Nutrition*, Oct. 2001; accessed Oct. 28, 2008, http://www.ajcn.org/cgi/content/abstract/74/4/549

Chandel, Amar. "Sweet Poison," *The Tribune Spectrum,* Mar. 14, 2004; accessed Mar. 22, 2005, http://www.tribuneindia.com/2004/20040314/spectrum/main1.htm

"Cholesterol and Heart Disease." Pcrm.org; accessed Oct. 25, 2008, http://www.pcrm.org/health/prevmed/chol_heartdisease.html

Christian, Chris. "Increase Testosterone Levels." Suite101.com, Nov.11, 2007; accessed Nov. 1, 2008, http://fitness.suite101.com/article.cfm/boost_your_testosterone_levels

Cichoke, Anthony J., DC. *Enzymes & Enzyme Therapy: How to Jump Start Your Way to Lifelong Good Health.* New Canaan: Keats Publishing Inc., 1994.

Coates, C. David. *Old MacDonalds Factory Farm.* New York: The Continuum Publishing Co., 1989.

"Coffee May Be Linked to Rheumatoid Arthritis." Sciencedaily.com, July 2000; accessed Nov. 25, 2008, http://www.sciencedaily.com/releases/2000/07/000727080902.htm

Cohen, Robert. *Essence of Betrayal,* accessed March 1, 2005, http://www.notmilk.com/forum/594.html

Collingwood, Jane. "Emotions and Weight Affect Testosterone Levels." Psychcentral.com, Jan. 8, 2007; accessed Nov. 1, 2008, http://psychcentral.com/lib/2007/emotions-and-weight-affect-testosterone-levels/

"Common Dairy Digestive Under-Recognized and Under-Diagnosed in Minorities." Johnson & Johnson, accessed Feb. 13, 2005, http://www.jnj.com/news/jnj_news/20020311_0944.htm

Cook, Christopher D. "Environmental Hogwash: The EPA works with factory farms to delay regulation of 'Extremely Hazardous Substances.'" Oct. 6, 2004; accessed Jan. 27, 2005, http://www.inthesetimes.com/site/main/print/environmental_hogwash/

Cotterchio M, Boucher BA, Manno M, Gallinger S, Okey AB, Harper. "Red Meat Again Linked to Colorectal Cancer." Pcrm.org, received by e-mail; accessed Nov. 7, 2008

Coupe, Kevin. "Editorial: Mad Cows, Lunatic Politicians, & The Case for Traceback." Cattlenetwork.com, May 1, 2006; accessed Sept. 9, 2007, http://www.cattlenetwork.com/content.asp?contentid=33332

Cousens, Gabriel MD. *Conscious Eating.* Berkeley: North Atlantic Books, 2000.

Cousin, Jean Pierre, and Kirsten Hartvig. *Vitality Foods for Health and Fitness.* London: Duncan Baird, 2002.

Sources

"Dairy Products Linked to Prostate Cancer." Health Professionals follow-up study. Associated Press, April 5, 2000

Dale, Mary Claire. "Equal, Splenda Settle Lawsuit Over Ad Claims." Splendaexposed.com, May 15, 2007; accessed Nov. 29, 2008

Davis, Gail. "A Tale of Two Sweeteners: Aspartame & Stevia," accessed Feb. 12, 2005, http://suewidemark.netfirms.com/davis.htm

Delany, Richard M., MD, FACC, "Omega-3 Fat During Pregnancy." DrDelany.com, accessed March 6, 2006, http://www.drdelany.com/Preventive_Updates_2004_test_51.asp?patient=

Des Maisons, Kathleen, PhD. *Potatoes Not Prozac.* New York: Fireside, 1998.

Diamond, Harvey, and Marilyn Diamond. *Fit for Life.* New York: Warner, 1985.

Diamond, Harvey, and Marilyn Diamond. *Fit for Life II: Living Health.* New York: Warner, 1987.

"Diet and Alzheimer's Disease." Pcrm.org, Aug. 11, 2004; accessed Nov. 20, 2008, http://www.pcrm.org/health/prevmed/diet_alzheimers.html

Djousse L, Gaziano JM, Buring JE, Lee I. "Egg Consumption Linked to Risk of Type 2 Diabetes." Pcrm.org, sent as e-mail Nov 23, 2008.

Dorfman, Lisa MS, RD, LMHC. *The Vegetarian Sports Nutrition Guide.* New York: John Wiley & Sons, Inc. 2000.

"Drug-Resistant Bacteria Found in U.S. Meat." *Reuters Medical News,* May 24, 2001.

"E. Coli Infection." Familydoctor.org, *American Academy of Family Physicians*, updated Sept 2006; accessed Sept. 9, 2007, http://familydoctor.org/242.xml

"Eggs Non Gratis." *The Civil Abolitionist,* autumn 2008, accessed Mar. 13, 2007, http://web.linkny.com/~civitas/page74.html

Eisnitz, Gail A. "Ask the Experts." Peta.org, accessed March 17, 2005, http://www.goveg.com/vegkit/meet.asp

Eisnitz, Gail A. *Slaughterhouse: The Shocking Story of Greed, Neglect, and Inhumane Treatment Inside the U.S. Meat Industry.* Amherst: Prometheus Books, 1997.

Epstein, Samuel, S., MD. *The Politics of Cancer (Revisited)*, East Ridge Press, NY, 1998

Esselstyn, Caldwell B., Jr., MD. *Prevent and Reverse Heart Disease.* New York: Avery, 2008.

"Factory Farming: Environmental Consequences." Animalalliance.ca, accessed March 29, 2005, http://www.animalalliance.ca/kids/facfar1.htm#environment

"Fact vs. Fiction." Truthaboutsplenda.com, accessed Feb. 14, 2005, http://www.truthaboutsplenda.com/factvsfiction/index.html>

Farlow, Christine Hoza, DC. *Food Additives: A Shopper's Guide to What's Safe & What's Not.* Escondido: KISS for Health, 2004.

"FDA Approved Animal Drug Products." FDA "Green Book" section, accessed March 21, 2005, http://dil.vetmed.vt.edu/NadaFirst/NADA.cfm

Ferdowsian, Hope, MD, MPH, e-mail to Rory Freedman, December 1, 2008.

Ferdowsian, Hope, MD, MPH and Susan Levin, RD. "Fish Still Not a Healthy Choice." *The Providence Journal,* Oct. 24, 2006; accessed Nov. 21, 2006, http://www.pcrm.org/news/commentary061024.html

Sources

"Fish and Shellfish: Contamination Problems Preclude Inclusion in the Dietary Guidelines for Americans." Pcrm.org, spring 2004, accessed March 31, 2005, http://www.pcrm.org/health/reports/fish_report.html>

"Fish Feel Pain." Fishinghurts.com., accessed March 3, 2005, http://www.fishinghurts.com/FishFeelPain.asp

"5 Ways to Boost Your Testosterone Levels." Healthandmen.com, Aug. 11, 2007; accessed Nov. 29, 2008, http://www.healthandmen.com/2007/08/11/5-ways-to-boost-your-testosterone-levels/

"Food Additives." New-fitness.com, accessed Feb. 4, 2005, http://www.new-fitness.com/nutrition/food_additives.html

"Food and Nutrition Assistance Programs." Economic Research Service, U.S. Department of Agriculture, USDA.gov; updated March 18, 2005; accessed March 22, 2005, http://www.ers.usda.gov/Briefing/FoodNutritionAssistance/

Fox, Mary Kay, William Hamilton, and Biing-Hwan Lin. "Effects of Food Assistance and Nutrition Programs on Nutrition and Health: Volume 4, Executive Summary of the Literature Review." USDA economicresearchservice.gov, Dec. 2004; accessed Nov. 22, 2008, http://ers.usda.gov/publications/fanrr19-4/

"Free-Range Eggs and Meat: Conning Consumers?" Peta.org, accessed March 16, 2005, http://www.peta.org/mc/factsheet_display.asp?ID=96

Friedrich, Bruce. e-mail to Rory Freedman, December 19, 2008.

Friedrich, Bruce. "Taking the Food Crisis Personally." Huffingtonpost.com, June 20, 2008; accessed Jan. 11, 2009, http://www.huffingtonpost.com/bruce-friedrich/taking-the-food-crisis-pe_b _107992.html

Friedrich, Bruce. "Why Not Give a Vegetarian Diet a Try for the New Year?" huffingtonpost.com, Dec. 30, 2007; accessed Jan. 11, 2009, http://www.huffingtonpost.com/bruce-friedrich/why-not-give-a-vegetarian_ b_78805.html

Fuhrman, Joel, MD. *Eat to Live.* Boston, New York, London: Little, Brown, 2003.

Gates, Donna. *The Body Ecology Diet*, accessed Feb. 25, 2005, http://www.holisticmed.com/sweet/stv-cook.txt

Gelles, Jeff. "Why antibiotics in meat should give you pause." *The Philadelphia Inquirer.* Dec. 11, 2002.

Giovannucci E, Rimm E, Wolk A, et al. "Calcium and Fructose Intake in Relation to Risk of Prostate Cancer." Cancer Res 1998a; 58:442-7.

Giovannucci, E. "Dietary influences of 1, 25 (OH)2 vitamin D in relation to prostate cancer: a hypothesis." Cancer Causes and Control 9 (1998): 567-582.

Giovannucci, E, Eric B. Rimm, Meir J. Stampfer, Graham A. Colditz, Alberto Ascherio, and Walter C. Willett. "Intake of Fat, Meat and Fiber in Relation to Risk of Colon Cancer in Men." *American Association for Cancer Research*, May 1994; accessed Nov. 22, 2008, http://cancerres.aacrjournals.org/cgi/content/abstract/54/9/2390

Giovannucci E., et al., "Tomatoes, Tomato-Based Products, Lycopene, and Cancer: Review of the epidemiologic literature," *Journal of the National Cancer Institute*, 91 (1999): 317-31.

Sources

Gold, Mark. Aspartame Toxicity Info Center article, "Formaldehyde Poisoning from Aspartame," Dec. 9, 1998; accessed March 6, 2005, http://www.holisticmed.com/aspartame/embalm.html

Gold, Mark. "Aspartame/NutraSweet Toxicity Summary." Nov. 30, 2000; accessed March 3, 2005, http://www.holisticmed.com/aspartame/summary.html

Gold, Mark. "Common Toxic and Unhealthy Substances to Avoid," accessed Feb. 28, 2005, http://www.holisticmed.com/aspartame/history.faq

Gold, Mark. "Scientific Abuse in Methanol/Formaldehyde Research Related to Aspartame," accessed Jan. 12, 2005, http://www.holisticmed.com/aspartame/abuse/methanol.html

Gold, Mark. "Toxicity Effects of Aspartame Use," accessed Feb. 2, 2005, http://www.holisticmed.com/aspartame/

Gold, Mark. "The Bitter Truth about Artificial Sweeteners." Truth Campaign; accessed March 23, 2005, http://www.ivanfrasier.com

Gottlieb, Scott. "High-protein diet brings risk of kidney stones." BMJ.com, Aug. 24, 2002; accessed Dec. 4, 2008, http://www.bmj.com/cgi/content/full/325/7361/408/d

Grace, Matthew. *A Way Out: Dis-Ease Deception and The Truth About Health*. U.S.A: Matthew Grace, 2000.

"The Great Sugar Debate: Is It Vegan?" accessed Feb. 20, 2005, http://www.vegfamily.com/articles/sugar.htm

Greger, Michael, MD. "Rocket Fuel in Milk," accessed Jan. 23, 2005, http://all-creatures.org/health/rocket.html

Green, Che. "Not Milk: The USDA, Monsanto, and the U.S. Dairy Industry."

LiP Magazine, July 9, 2002; accessed Feb. 20, 2005,
http://www.alternet.org/story/13557/

Grogan, Bryanna Clark. "A Few Words About Sugar and Other Sweeteners,"
accessed Feb. 22, 2005,
http://www.vegsource.com/articles/bryanna_sugar.htm

"Growing and Processing Sugar." The Sugar Association; accessed Jan. 12,
2005, http://www.sugar.org/facts/grow.html

Halliday, Jess. "Study links low sperm with high soy consumption."
Foodnavigator.com, Jul. 24, 2008; accessed Nov. 24, 2008,
http://www.foodnavigator.com/layout/set/print/Product-Categories/Protein
s-non-dairy/Study-links-low-sperm-with-high-soy-consumption

Harris, Simon. "Organic Consumers Association (OCA) Denounces
Degradation of Organic Food Standards by Congress," accessed Feb. 10,
2005, http://environment.about.com/library/pressrelease/bloca.htm

Hasselberger, Sepp. "Aspartame: RICO Complaint Filed Against NutraSweet,
ADA, Monsanto." Sept. 17, 2004; accessed Feb. 15, 2005,
http://www.newmediaexplorer.org/sepp/2004/09/17/aspartame_rico_compl
aint_filed_against_nutrasweet_ada_monsanto.htm>

Hatherill, Robert J., PhD. *Eat to Beat Cancer*. Los Angeles: Renaissance
Books, 1998.

"Health Concerns About Dairy Products." Pcrm.org; accessed Dec. 5, 2008,
http://pcrm.org/health/veginfo/dairy.html

Healthy Child Online Articles and Resources, accessed March 2, 2005,
http://www.healthychild.com/database/life_is_sweet_a_guide_to_using_he
althy_sweeteners.htm

Sources

"The Hidden Lives of Chickens," accessed March 3, 2005,
http://www.peta.org/feat/hiddenlives/

"High Blood Pressure." American Hearth Association; accessed Dec. 5, 2008,
http://www.americanheart.org/presenter.jhtml?identifier=4623

"High Blood Pressure (Hypertension)." Pcrm.org; accessed Oct. 25, 2008,
http://www.pcrm.org/health/prevmed/high_blood_pressure.html

Holford, Patrick. *The Optimum Nutrition Bible*. Berkeley: The Crossing Press,
1999.

Hooper, Lee, Rachel L. Thompson, Roger A. Harrison, Carolyn D.
Summerbell, Andy R Ness, Helen J. Moore, Helen V. Worthington, Paul
N. Durrington, Julian P. T. Higgins, Nigel E. Capps, Rudolph A.
Riemersma, Shah B. J. Ebrahim, and George Davey Smith.

"Human Physiology." Goveg.com, accessed Dec. 5, 2008,
http://www.goveg.com/naturalhumandiet_physiology.asp

"How Can I Get Enough Protein? The Protein Myth." PCRM.org; accessed
Nov. 15, 2008, http://www.pcrm.org/health/veginfo/protein.html

"How Exercise Reduces Your Risk of Prostate Cancer." Mercola.com, May 26,
2005; accessed Dec. 5, 2008,
http://articles.mercola.com/sites/articles/archive/2005/05/26/exercise-cance
r-part-four.aspx

Howell, Edward MD. *Enzyme Nutrition: The Food Enzyme Concept*. U.S.A.:
Avery, 1985.

Howell, Laurie. "#193 Why Choose Organic Coffee?" accessed Feb. 25, 2005,
http://www.thegreenscene.com/shows/193.html

Hull, Dr. Janet Starr. *Splenda: is it safe or not?* Dallas, TX: The Pickle Press, 2004

"The Importance of Water for Athletes" Fitsense.com; accessed Dec.5, 2008,
http://www.fitsense.co.uk/fit_article.php?id=81

"In Men, Exercise Benefits Prostate, Sexuality." Medicalnewstoday.com, May
7, 2007; accessed Nov. 26, 2008,
http://www.medicalnewstoday.com/printerfriendlynews.php?newsid=70057

Incident Heart Failure Is Associated with Lower Whole-Grain Intake and
Greater High-Fat Dairy and Egg Intake in the Atherosclerosis Risk in
Communities (ARIC) Study, *Journal of the American Dietetic Association,*
Volume 108, Issue 11, Pages 1881-1887 (November 2008)

"Investigation Reveals Slaughter Horrors at Agriprocessors." Peta.org,
accessed March 17, 2005, http://www.goveg.com/feat/agriprocessors/

Johnson, Lucy. "Aspartame . . . A Killer!" *The Sunday Express London, U.K.*
Newfrontier.com; accessed March 21, 2005,
http://www.newfrontier.com/asheville/aspartame.htm

Jolley, Chuck. "Hallmark/Westland Might Not Be An Anomaly According To
An OIG Report," CattleNetwork.com; accessed Jan. 9, 2009,
http://www.cattlenetwork.com/Content.asp?ContentID=275451

Jones, Lisa. "Spray n' Wash: Go organic and boost testosterone levels."
Menshealth.com; accessed Nov. 29, 2008,
http://www.menshealth.com/cda/article.do?site=MensHealth&channel=s
ex.relationships&conitem=96d506d667b4a010VgnVCM100000cfe793cd

Kamen, Betty, PhD. *New Facts About Fiber.* Novato: Nutrition Encounter,
1991.

Katcher, Joshua, "Lean & Green: Jake Shields." Thediscerningbrute.com;

Sources

accessed Nov. 23, 2008,
http://thediscerningbrute.com/2008/11/05/jake-shields/

Keri, Jonah. "Who says you have to eat meat to be a successful athlete?"
ESPNthemag.com, updated July 22, 2008; accessed Nov. 10, 2008
http://sports.espn.go.com/espn/page2/story?page=keri/080616&sportCat=
mlb

Kirchheimer, Sid. "High-Protein Diets Can Hurt Kidneys: Damage Stems from
Proteins Found in Meat." Webmd.com, Mar. 17, 2003; accessed Dec. 5,
2008,
http://www.webmd.com/news/20030317/high-protein-diets-can-hurt-kidneys

Krebs, A.V. "USDA Accused of Allowing 'Sham Certifiers' into the National
Organic Program." *The Agribusiness Examiner.* Issue #367, Aug. 23, 2004;
accessed Jan. 25, 2005, http://www.organicconsumers.org/organic/usda.cfm

Krumm, Susan. "Refining process has sweet ending." Lawrence Journal-World,
June 13, 2001; accessed Jan. 20, 2005,
http://ljworld.com/section/cookingqa/story/55875

Larson-Meyer, D. Enette, PhD, RD. *Vegetarian Sports Nutrition.* Champaign,
IL: Human Kinetics 2007.

Langeland, Terje. Tainted Meat, Tainted Money: Consumer Groups Decry
Coziness Between Government, Agribusiness." *Colorado Springs
Independent* online edition, Aug. 1-7, 2002; accessed Feb. 20, 2005,
http://www.csindy.com/csindy/2002-08-01/cover2.html

Langley, Gill, MA, PhD. *Vegan Nutrition: A Survey of Research.* Oxford: The
Vegan Society, 1988.

"The Latest in Cancer: 'White Meat' Linked to Colon Cancer." Pcrm.org,

winter 1999; accessed Mar. 28, 2005,
http://www.pcrm.org/magazine/GM99Winter9.html

Leake, Jonathon. "The rich and emotional lives of cows." News.com; accessed Feb. 28, 2005,
http://www.news.com/au/story/0,10117,12390397-13762,00.html

"Livestock a major threat to the environment." Fao.org, Nov. 29, 2006; accessed Sept. 9, 2007,
http://www.fao.org/newsroom/en/news/2006/1000448/index.html

Lorenzi, Rossella, "Study: Chickens Think About Future," animal.discovery.com; accessed January 7, 2009,
http://animal.discovery.com/news/briefs/20050711/chicken.html

"Lycopene: Benefits, Side Effects, Sources and Supplements," Health.learninginfo.org; accessed Dec. 9, 2008,
http://health.learninginfo.org/lycopene-benefits.htm

Mason, Jim, and Peter Singer. *Animal Factories.* New York: Crown, 1990.

Martin, Andrew, "How to Add Oomph to 'Organic'," *The New York Times*, Aug. 19, 2007; accessed Sept. 9, 2007,
http://www.nytimes.com/2007/08/19/business/yourmoney/19feed.html?ex=1189310400&en=2b9b40776ea0c111&ei=5070

McCaleb, Rob. "Stevia Leaf—Too Good to Be Legal?" Herb Research Foundation, accessed Feb. 14, 2005,
http://www.holisticmed.com/sweet/stv-faq.txt

McDougall, John. M.D. "Saving Yourself From Prostate (or Breast) Cancer." Vegsource.com; accessed Nov. 1, 2008, March 1999; accessed Sept. 9, 2007,
http://findarticles.com/p/articles/mi_m0NAH/is_2_29/ai_53929987

Sources

"McNeil Nutritionals and Sugar Association Settle Splenda Suit." *Philadelphia Business Journal*, Nov. 17, 2008; accessed Dec. 5, 2008, http://philadelphia.bizjournals.com/philadelphia/stories/2008/11/17/daily13.html

McPhatter, MS, RD, CSR. "Too Much of a Good Thing: Limiting Protein Intake in Chronic Kidney Disease." Aakp.org: accessed Dec. 5, 2008, http://www.aakp.org/aakp-library/Limiting-Protein-Intake/

"*Men's Health* Warns of Foods You Should Never Eat." Peta.org, accessed March 23, 2005, http://www.peta.org/feat/menshealth/

Mercola, Joseph, MD, with Alison Rose Levy. *The No-Grain Diet: Conquer Carbohydrate Addiction and Stay Slim for Life.* New York: Dutton, 2003.

Mercola, Joseph, MD. "The Secret Dangers of Splenda (Sucralose), an Artificial Sweetener," Dec. 3, 2000; accessed Feb. 20, 2005, http://www.mercola.com/2000/dec/3/sucralose_dangers.htm#

Mercola, Joseph, MD. "Splenda—Here We Go Again." July 21, 2004; accessed Feb. 12, 2005, http://www.mercola.com/fcgi/pf/2004/jul/21/splenda.htm

Mercola, Joseph, MD. "US 'Food Pyramid' Invalid as It Was Made by Experts with Conflicts of Interest." Nov. 19, 2000; accessed Jan. 10, 2005, http://www.mercola.com/2000/nov/19/food_pyramid.htm

"Milk Sucks." Peta.org.; milksucks.com, accessed March 12, 2005, http://www.milksucks.com/

Mills, Dixie J. MD, FACS. "Health benefits of soy—why the controversy?" Womentowomen.com, last modified Mar. 9, 2007; accessed Mar. 21, 2007, http://www.womentowomen.com/nutritionandweight-loss/healthbenefitsofsoy.asp

Mills, Milton R, MD. "The Comparative Anatomy of Eating," Vegsource.org, accessed Dec 5, 2008 http://www.vegsource.com/veg_faq/comparative.htm

Mindell, Earl R., PhD, with Hester Mundis. *Earl Mindells New Vitamin Bible*. New York, Boston: Warner, 2004.

"Molasses." Oct. 2, 2003; accessed Feb. 2, 2005, http://www.everything2.com/index.pl?node=molasses

"Molasses nutrition data." accessed March 3, 2005, http://www.nutritiondata.com/facts-001-02s04at.html

Moore, Heather. "Vegetarian Athletes: At the Top of Their Game." Gather.com, Feb. 4, 2008; accessed Nov. 20, 2008, http://www.gather.com/viewArticle.jsp?articleId=281474977249417

Murray, Lynda MA, RD, LD, CSSD. "Lots to watch out for on a high protein diet." Nashuatelegraph.com, Nov 19, 2008; accessed Dec 5, 2008,

http://www.nashuatelegraph.com/apps/pbcs.dll/article?AID=/20081119/COLU MNISTS44/811189917/-1/food

Murray, Rich. "How Aspartame Became Legal-The Timeline." Dec. 24, 2002; accessed March 5, 2005, http://www.quantumbalancing.com/news/aspartameapproved.htm

Myss, Caroline, PhD. *Anatomy of the Spirit: The Seven Stages of Power and Healing*. New York: Three Rivers Press, 1996.

"National Cattlemans Beef Association Pays for Sadistic Anti-Vegan 'Study.'" Vegsource Interactive Inc., accessed Feb. 22, 2005, http://www.vegsource.com/articles2/ncbs_vegan_study.htm

"National School Lunch Program Background," healthyschoollunches.org, accessed Jan. 11, 2009,

Sources

http://www.healthyschoollunches.org/background/commodity.html

"National Soft Drink Association Protest (Summary)." Congressional Record-Senate, March 11, 2005; accessed Jan. 20, 2005, http://www.dorway.com/nsda.txt

Nations Largest Organic Dairy Brand, Horizon, Accused of Violating Organic Standards. The Cornucopia Institute, Feb. 16, 2005, http://www.cornucopia.org, Mar. 2, 2005, http://www.organicconsumers.org/organic/horizon21705.cfm

"Natural Sweeteners." Natural Nutrition, accessed Feb. 2, 2005, http://www.livrite.com/sweeten.htm

Natural Sweetener-Safe for Diabetics," accessed Feb. 15, 2005, http://www.primalnature.com/stevia.html

Ness, Carol. "Organic Food: Outcry Over Rule Changes that Allow More Pesticides, Hormones. *The San Francisco Chronicle*, May 22, 2004, accessed Mar. 2, 2005; http://www.commondreams.org/cgi-bin/print.cgi?file=/headlines04/0522-09.htm

Nestle, Marion. *Food Politics: How the Food Industry Influences Nutrition and Health*. California: University of California, 2000, 2007.

"New Study Shows Being Fit Lowers Risk for Stroke." Menwell.com, Apr. 27, 2008; accessed Nov. 25, 2008, http://www.menwell.com.au/news/new-study-shows-being-fit-lowers-risk-for-stroke/

Notmilk.com. March 5, 2005, http://notmilk.com/forum/526.html

Nutt, Amy Ellis. "In the Soil, Water, Food, Air." *The Star-Ledger*, Dec. 8, 2000.

"OCA and Environmental Groups Sue USDA to Enforce Strict Standards:

Environmental Groups Back Harvey Lawsuit." *Organic Business News*, Dec. 2004, vol. 16, no. 12; accessed Jan. 12, 2005, http://organicconsumers.org/organic/lawsuit010505.cfm

"Omega-3 Fatty Acids." Umm.edu, reviewed May 1, 2007; accessed Dec. 6, 2008, http://www.umm.edu/altmed/articles/omega-3-000316.htm

"Organic Industry and Consumers Celebrate USDA Reversal on Non-Food National Organic Standards" press release, May 26, 2004; accessed Feb. 10, 2005, http://www.westonaprice.org/federalupdate/aa2004/infoalert_052604.html

Ornish, Dean, M.D. *Eat More, Weigh Less*. New York: Harper Collins, 2001.

Osborne, Sally Eauclaire. "Does Soy Have a Dark Side?" *Natural Health*, March 1999; accessed Sept. 9, 2007, http://findarticles.com/p/articles/mi_m0NAH/is_2_29/ai_53929987

"Osteoporosis Men." Nof.org; accessed Nov. 29, 2008, http://www.nof.org/men/

Parrish, Michael. "Famous Olympic Wrestler Sushil Kumar Promotes Vegetarian Lifestyle with PETA." Ecorazzi.com; accessed Nov. 13, 2008 http://www.ecorazzi.com/2008/11/13/famous-olympic-wrestler-sushil-kumar-promotes-vegetarian-lifestyle-with-peta/

Pert, Candace B., PhD. *Molecules of Emotion*. New York: Scribner, 1997.

"Pigs: Smart Animals at the Mercy of the Pork Industry." Peta.org, accessed March 3, 2005, http://www.peta.org.factsheet/files/FactsheetDisplay.asp?ID=119

"Protein: Moving Closer to Center Stage." Harvard.edu; accessed Mar. 13, 2007, http://www.hsph.harvard.edu/nutritionsource/what-should-you-eat/protein

Sources

-full-story/index.html

Pyevich, Caroline. "Sugar and other sweeteners: Do they contain animal products?" *Vegetarian Journal*, volume XVI, no. 2, Mar./Apr. 1997; accessed Feb. 25, 2005, http://www.stanford.edu/group/vegan/sweetners.htm

Quinn, Elizabeth. "Water Intoxication-Hyponatremia: Can Athletes Drink Too Much Water?" About.com, Feb. 25, 2008; accessed Dec. 1, 2008, http://sportsmedicine.about.com/od/hydrationandfluid/a/Hyponatremia.htm

Ralston, Katherine.; Constance Newman.; Annette Clauson.; Joanne Guthrie.; Jean Buzby. "The National School Lunch Program Background, Trends, and Issues." USDA, July 18, 2008; accessed Nov. 22, 2008, http://ers.usda.gov/Publications/ERR61/

"Reduce Heart Disease Risk: Encourage and Prescribe Exercise for Your Patients." Medscape.com, Feb. 26, 2004; accessed Dec. 4, 2008, www.medscape.com/viewarticle/470115

"Ricky Williams is a vegetarian professional NFL football player." Happycow.net; accessed Nov. 25, 2008, http://www.happycow.net/famous/ricky_williams/

Riley, Laura, MD, OB/GYN, and Stacey Nelson, MS, RD, LDN. *You and Your Baby: Healthy Eating During Pregnancy. Your Guide to Eating Well and Staying Fit*. Iowa: Meredith Books, 2006

"Risks and benefits of omega-3 fats for mortality, cardiovascular disease, and cancer: systemic review." *British Medical Journal*, 2006; 332: 752-760 (Apr. 1) Mar. 24, 2006; accessed Sept. 11, 2007, http://www.bmj.com/cgi/content/full/332/7544/752?ehom

Robbins, John. *Diet for a New America*. Walpole: Stillpoint, 1987.

Robbins, John. *The Food Revolution: How Your Diet Can Help Save Your Life and Our World*. San Francisco, CA: Conari Press, 2001.

Robbins, John. "What About Soy?" Foodrevolution.org; accessed Mar. 1, 2007, http://www.foodrevolution.org/what_about_soy.htm

Roberts, H. J., MD. "The Bressler Report." *Sun Sentinel Press*; accessed Feb. 22, 2005, http://www.presidiotex.com/bressler/

"Salmon farms producing tainted fish-farmed salmon not as healthy as wild salmon and fish farming industry pollutes the ocean." *The New York Times*. May 28, 2003; accessed Sept. 9, 2007, http://www.findarticles.com/p/articles/mi_m0876/is_86/ai_111303246

"Salts That Heal and Salts That Kill." Curezone.com, accessed March 14, 2005, http://www.curezone.com/foods/saltcure.asp

Savona, Natalie. *The Kitchen Shrink: Foods and Recipes for a Healthy Mind*. London: Duncan Baird, 2003.

Saxe, Gordon MD, PhD. "Ask the Doctor." *Cancer Project*, summer 2006; accessed Dec.5, 2007, www.cancerproject.org/media/newsletter/jul06/ask.php

Scala, James, PHD., *25 Natural Ways to Lower Blood Pressure*. New York: McGraw Hill, 2002.

Schlosser, Eric. "The Cow Jumped Over the U.S.D.A." *The New York Times*, Jan. 2, 2004; accessed Mar. 1, 2005, http://www.commondreams.org/views04/0102-06.htm

Schlosser, Eric. *Fast Food Nation: The Dark Side of the All-American Meal*. New York: Perennial, 2002.

Schnitzer, Dr. Johann Georg. "History of the Human Diet." Alive.com, May

Sources

2003; accessed Nov. 23, 2008,
http://www.alive.com/1338a4a2.php?subject_bread_cramb=463

Severson, Kim. "Dairy Council to End Ad Campaign That Linked Drinking Milk With Weight Loss." *NY Times* on the web May 11, 2007; accessed Jan. 9, 2009, http://www.nytimes.com/2007/05/11/us/11milk.html

Severson, Kim. "Sugar coated: Were drowning in high fructose corn syrup. Do the risks go beyond our waistline?" *San Francisco Chronicle*, Feb. 18, 2004; accessed Feb. 10, 2005,
http://www.sfgate.com/cgi-bin/article.cgi?f=/chronicle/archive/2004/02/18/FDGS24VKMH1.DTL

Sherman, Janette D., MD, *Life's Delicate Balance*, Taylor & Francis, NY, 2000.

"Silent Spring II." Thirdworldtraveler.com, from the summer 1997 *Food First Newsletter*, accessed Mar. 6, 2007,
http://www.thirdworldtraveler.com/Environment/Silent_Spring2.html

Simon, Michele. "Dairy Industry Propaganda: Tale of Two Mega-Campaigns." Originally published at Vegan.com, April 1999; accessed Feb. 7, 2005,
http://www.informedeating.org/docs/dairy_industry_propaganda.html

Simon, Michele. "Misery on the Menu: The National School Lunch Program." Originally published in *The Animals Agenda*, September/October 1998; accessed Feb. 7, 2005,
http://www.informedeating.org/docs/misery_on_the_menu.html

Simon, Michele, JD, MPH. "The Politics of Meat and Dairy," accessed Jan. 26, 2005, http://wwwearthsave.org/news/polsmd.htm

Squires, Sally. "Sweet but Not So Innocent?" *The Washington Post*, Mar. 11, 2003; accessed Feb. 18, 2005,
http://www.washingtonpost.com/ac2/wp-dyn/A8003-2003Mar10?language

=printer

Steinman, David. *Diet For a Poisoned Planet: How to Choose Safe Foods for You and Your Family*. New York: Harmony, 1990.

Steinman, David. *Diet For a Poisoned Planet: How to Choose Safe Foods for You and Your Family: the Twenty-First Century Edition.* New York: Thunder's Mouth Press, 2007.

Sternberg, Holly. Rev. of *The Body Restoration Plan* by Paula Baillie-Hamilton MD, and Rev. of *Animal Factories* by Jim Mason and Peter Singer; Aug. 17, 2003; accessed Mar. 8, 2005, http://groups.yahoo.com/group/AnimalAdvocacy/message/3487

"Soft Drinks, High-Fructose Corn Syrup Promote Diabetes, Says Study." March 10, 2005; accessed March 15, 2005, http://www.newstarget.com/002584

Stolzenberg-Solomon, Rachel, Amanda J. Cross, Debra T. Silverman, Catherine Schairer, Frances E. Thompson, Victor Kipnis, Amy F. Subar, Albert Hollenbeck, Arthur Schatzkin, and Rashmi Sinha. "Meat and Meat-Mutagen Intake and Pancreatic Cancer Risk in the NIH-AARP Cohort." *American Association for Cancer Research*, Dec. 1, 2007; accessed Nov. 22, 2008, http://cebp.aacrjournals.org/cgi/content/abstract/16/12/2664

"Sugar Blues." Natural Nutrition, accessed Feb. 2, 2005, http://livrite.com/sugar1.htm>

"Summary List of Vegan/Vegetarian." Veganathlete.com; accessed Dec.1, 2008 http://www.veganathlete.com/vegan_vegetarian_athletes.php

"Surgeon General Asks: Got Bones?" Gotmilk.com, Oct. 26, 2004; accessed March 21, 2005, http://www.gotmilk.com/news/news_035.html

Sources

"10 Reasons to Avoid Acidosis." Poly MVA Survisors.com; accessed Mar. 28, 2005, http://polymvasurvivors.com/4corners_coral.html

"Top 10 Reasons Not to Eat Chickens." Goveg.com; accessed Mar. 13, 20007, http://www.goveg.com/f-top10chickens.asp

"Toxic Shock." Goveg.com; accessed Mar. 13, 2007, http://goveg.com/contamination.asp

"3/4 Chickens Bought Nationwide Harbor Salmonella or Campylobacter." Organicconsumers.org. *Consumer Reports* Jan 2003; accessed Mar. 13, 2007, http://www.organicconsumers.org/toxic/chixyuck.cfm

"Two New Studies Sour Milk's Image." Pcrm.org, Dec. 3, 2004; accessed March 20, 2005, http://www.pcrm.org/news/release041202.html

"Unhealthy link between caffeine and diabetes." *CBC Health & Science News*, Jan. 9, 2002; accessed Feb. 20, 2005, http://www.cbc.ca/story/science/national/2002/01/09/caffeine_diabetes020109.html

"Union of Concerned Scientists Food & Farming Newsletter." Organicconsumers.org, April 2006; accessed Sept. 9, 2007, http://organicconsumers.org/politics/FEED060417.cfm

"The U.S. Food and Drug Administration (FDA) and the glutamate industry." July 12, 2004; accessed Feb. 4, 2005, http://www.truthinlabeling.org/legislators2.html

"USDA wont stop use of illegal hormones in the veal industry: cancer rates skyrocket in humans." Jan. 26, 2005; accessed Jan. 27, 2005, http://www.newstarget.com/z0001067.html

U.S. Department of Agriculture. APIS Veterinary Services. January 2005. "National Animal Identification System: Goal and Vision"; accessed

March 12, 2005,
http://animalid.usda.gov/nais/about/nais_overview_factsheet.shtml

U.S. Department of Agriculture. "About USDA." Accessed March 12, 2005,
http://www.usda.gov/wps/portal/!ut/p/_s.7_0_A/7_0_1OB?navtype=MA&n
avid=ABOUT_USDA

U.S. Department of Health and Human Services. "Symptoms Attributed to
Aspartame in Complaints Submitted to the FDA." April 20, 1995; accessed
Feb. 22, 2005,
http://www.presidiotex.com/aspartame/Facts/92_Symptoms/92_symptoms.
html

Van Straten, Michael. *Super Detox.* London: Quadrille, 2003.

"USTR demands Japan lift beef import restrictions linked to cow age," *Japan
Today* online, accessed Sept. 15, 2007,
http://www.japantoday.com/jp/news/400520

"Vegetables Lower Prostate Cancer Risk," *Journal of the National Cancer
Institute* 92 (2000): 61-8, *Loma Linda University Vegetarian Nutrition and
Health Letter*, March 2000

"Vegan FAQs." *Vegan Action,* accessed Jan. 20, 2005,
http://www.vegan.org/FAQs/

"Vegan Ultimate Fighter Ricardo Moreira." Mmacoverage.com, Sept. 6, 2007;
accessed Nov. 28, 2008,
http://mmacoverage.com/vegan-ultimate-fighter-ricardo-moreira.html

"Vegetarian and Vegan Famous Athletes." Veggie.org, accessed March 21,
2005, http://veggie.org/veggie/famous.veg.athletes.shtml

"Vegetarian 101." GoVeg.com, accessed Oct. 18, 2008,

Sources

http://www.goveg.com/vegetarian101.asp

Vincent, Beth, MHS. "The importance of DHA during pregnancy and breastfeeding." Pregnancyandbaby.com; accessed Sept. 9, 2007, http://pregnancyandbaby.com/pregnancy/baby/The-importance-of-DHA-d uring-pregnancy-and-breastfeeding-5726.htm

Waehner, Paige. "Exercise Bulimia, the New Eating Disorder," accessed March 5, 2005, http://exercise.about.com/cs/exercisehealth/ a/exercisebulimia_p.htm

Wangen, Stephen, ND. "Food Allergy Solutions Review." FoodAllergySolutions.com, July 2003; accessed March 28, 2005, http://www.foodallergysolutions.com/food-allergy-news0307.html

"What Men Should Know About Low Testosterone." Menshealthnetwork.org; accessed Nov. 29, 2008, http://www.menshealthnetwork.org/timeout/lowtestosterone.htm

Weil, Andrew, MD. *Natural Health, Natural Medicine*. Boston: Houghton Mifflin, 1998.

Weil, Andrew, MD. "Does Soy Have a Dark Side?" Dr. Andrew Weil's Self Healing, March 2003; accessed March 15, 2005, http://www.drweilselfhealing.com

Weiss, Suzanne E. *Readers Digest: Foods that Harm, Foods that Heal: An A-Z Guide to Safe and Healthy Eating*. Pleasantville: The Readers Digest Association Inc., 1997.

Whitney, Eleanor Noss, and Sharon Rady Rolfes. *Understanding Nutrition*, 8th ed. Belmont: Wadsworth, 1999.

Willet, Walter, et al., "Relation of Meat, Fat, and Fiber Intake to the Risk of

Colon Cancer," *New England Journal of Medicine*, Dec. 13, 1990; Willet quoted in Kolata, Gina "Animal Fat is Tied to Colon Cancer." *The New York Times*, Dec. 13, 1990.

Wijers-Hasegawa, Yumi. "Bayers GE Crop Herbicide, Glufosinate, Causes Brain Damage." Goldenharvestorganics.com, accessed March 28, 2005, http://www.ghorganics.com/COMMON%20PESTICIDE%20CAUSES%20AGGRESSION%20&%20BRAIN%20DAMAGE.htm

Williams, Rose Marie. "What's in the Beef? Interview with Howard Lyman, author of *Mad Cowboy*, Encyclopedia.com. Oct. 1, 2001; accessed Mar. 6, 2007, http://www.encyclopedia.com/doc/1G1-78900860.html

Young, Robert O. PhD., and Shelley Redford Young. *The pH Miracle: Balance Your Diet, Reclaim Your Health*. New York: Warner, 2002.

Endnotes

1 Steinman, *Diet for a Poisoned Planet*, 166-7

2 Cousens, *Conscious Eating,* 475.

3 Young, *The pH Miracle: Balance Your Diet, Reclaim Your Health,* 90.

4 Gold, "Aspartame Toxicity Info Center Article: Formaldehyde Poisoning from Aspartame."

5 Steinman, 190.

6 Ibid., 191.

7 "Caffeine," ecuremelife.com.

8 "Blood Pressure and Coffee Consumption, " menwell.com.au.

9 "Unhealthy link found between caffeine and diabetes," CBC Health & Science News.

10 "Coffee May Be Linked To Rheumatoid Arthritis," sciencedaily.com.

11 Young, 51.

12 Ibid., 24-5.

13 Howell, "Why Choose Organic Coffee?"

14 Steinman, 355.

15 Young, 75.

16 Pert, *Molecules of Emotion,* 321-22.

17 Ibid.

19 Whitney and Rolfes, *Understanding Nutrition*, 44.

20 Chandel, "Sweet Poison," *The Sunday Tribune Spectrum,* tribuneindia.com.

21 "Sugar Blues," Natural Nutrition, livrite.com.

22 Chandel.

23 "Soft Drinks, High-Fructose Corn Syrup Promote Diabetes, Says Study," newstarget.com.

24 "Natural Sweeteners," Natural Nutrition, livrite.com.

25 Gold, "Common Toxic and Substances to Avoid," holisticmed.com.

26 Ibid.

27 Ibid.

28 Ibid.

29 Murray, "How Aspartame Became

Legal-The Timeline,"
quantumbalancing.com.

30 Ibid.

31 Ibid.

32 "Department of Health and Human
Services Symptoms Attributed to
Aspartame in Complaints
Submitted to the FDA," U.S.
Department of Health and
Human Services,
presidiotex.com.

33 Johnson, "Aspartame . . . A Killer!"
The Sunday Express London,
newfrontier.com.

34 Hasselberger, "Aspartame: RICO
Complaint filed Against
Nutra-Sweet, ADA, Monsanto,"
newmediaexplorer.org.

35 Young, 89.

36 Gold, "The Bitter Truth about
Artificial Sweeteners,"
truthcampaign.ukf.net.

37 *Webster's New World Dictionary*
(1982), s.v. "saccharin."

38 Maryclaire Dale, "Equal, Splenda
Settle Lawsuit Over Ad Claims,"
splendaexposed.com.

39 Mercola, "The Secret Dangers of
Splenda (Sucralose), An
Artificial Sweetener,"
mercola.com.

40 Ibid., and Mercola,
"Splenda—Here We Go Again,"
mercola.com.

41 Ibid., "The Secret Dangers of
Splenda."

42 Burros, "Splenda's 'Sugar' Claim
Unites Odd Couple of Nutrition
Wars," *New York Times,*
skyhen.org.

43 Ibid.

44 "Equal, Splenda Settle Lawsuit
Over Ad Claims,"
splendaexposed.com.

45 Young, 50-51.

46 Ibid., 14-15.

47 Ibid.

48 Ibid.

49 Ibid.

50 "10 Reasons To Avoid Acidosis."

51 Young, 51-52.

52 Weil, *Natural Health, Natural
Medicine,* 27.

53 Murray, " Lots to watch out for on a
high-protein diet,"
nashuatelegraph.com.

54 Ibid.

55 Lesley L. McPhatter, MS, RD,
CSR, "Too Much of a Good
Thing: Limiting Protein Intake
in Chronic Kidney Disease."

Endnotes

Aakp.org.

[56] Scott Gottlieb, "High protein diet brings risk of kidney stones," bmj.com.

[57] Sid Kirchheimer, "High-Protein Diets Can Hurt Kidneys," webmd.com.

[58] Fuhrman, *Eat to Live,* 98.

[59] Ornish, Dean, M.D., *Eat More, Weigh Less,* xi.

[60] "Meat and Meat-Mutagen Intake and Pancreatic Cancer Risk in the NIH-AARP Cohort," cebp.aacrjounrals.org.

[61] "Cancer Prevention and Survival: Meat Consumption and Cancer Risk," cancerproject.org.

[62] "Intake of Fat, Meat, and Fiber in Relation to Risk of Colon Cancer in Men," cancererres.aacrjournals.org.

[63] Robbins, *The Food Revolution,* 49.

[64] "Red Meat Again Linked to Colorectal Cancer," pcrm.org.

[65] Campbell, *The China Study,* 168.

[66] "Intake of Fat, Meat, and Fiber in Relation to Risk of Colon Cancer in Men" and "Cancer Prevention and Survival: Cancer Facts—Colon Cancer," cancerproject.org and Campbell, *The China Study,* 237.

[67] Ibid., 95.

[68] Robbins, *Diet for a New America,* 290.

[69] "Diet and Alzheimer's Disease," pcrm.org.

[70] Schnitzer, "History of the Human Diet," alive.com.

[71] Grace, *A Way Out,* 8-9.

[72] Caldwell B. Esselstyn, Jr., M.D., *Prevent and Reverse Heart Disease,* 267.

[73] Grace, 8-10.

[74] Ibid.

[75] Ibid.

[76] Ibid.

[77] "Human Physiology," goveg.com.

[78] "Factory Farming," hfa.org.

[79] Gelles, "Why Antibiotics in Meat Should Give You Pause," *The Philadelphia Inquirer.*

[80] Cousens, *Conscious Eating,* 433.

[81] Steinman, 73.

[82] Ibid., 315.

[83] Ibid.

[84] Ibid.

[85] Ibid., 322.

[86] Ibid., 315.

[87] Hasegawa-Wijers, "Bayer's GE Crop Herbicide, Glufosinate, Causes Brain Damage."

[88] Associated Press, "Study Links Children's Asthma to Hog Farms."

[89] Steinman, *Diet for a New America* (21st century edition), 512.

[90] Ibid.

[91] Ibid.

[92] Ibid.

[93] Ibid.

[94] Ibid.

[95] Cousens, 438.

[96] Steinman, *Diet for a New America* (21st century edition)144-149.

[97] Ibid., 200-206.

[98] Ibid., 121.

[99] "Environmental Facts," kingwoodgreeninfo.org.

[100] Steinman, 80.

[101] "Men's Health Warns of Foods You Should Never Eat," Peta.org.

[102] Baillie-Hamilton, The Body Restoration Plan, 36.

[103] Ibid., 34-5.

[104] "FDA Approved Animal Drug Products," FDA "Green Book" section.

[105] Mason and Singer, Animal Factories, 75.

[106] Robbins, 303.

[107] "The Latest In Cancer: 'White Meat' Linked to Colon Cancer," pcrm.org; Singh PN, Fraser GE. Dietary risk factors for colon cancer in a low-risk population. *Am J Epidem* 1998; 148:761-74.

[108] Ibid.

[109] "Cancer Prevention and Survival: Meat Consumption and Cancer Risk," cancerproject.org.

[110] Steinman, 73.

[111] Ibid., 313-14.

[112] "Fish and Shellfish: Contamination Problems Preclude Inclusion in the Dietary Guidelines for Americans," pcrm.org, Spring 2004.

[113] Bruce Friedrich, "Why Not Give a Vegetarian Diet a Try for the New Year?" huffingtonpost.com.

[114] Diamond, *Fit For Life II,* 242.

[115] Cousens, 479.

[116] "10 Reasons To Avoid Acidosis," PolyMVASurvivors.com.

[117] Diamond, *Fit For Life II*, 243.

[118] "Health Concerns about Dairy Products" pcrm.org

Endnotes

119 Campbell and Campbell II, *The China Study,* 205.

120 Ibid., 204.

121 "Men and Osteoporosis," nof.org.

122 Ibid.

123 Campbell and Campbell II, 205.

124 Robbins, *Diet for a New America,* 164.

125 Watkins, "Dealing with Dairy Allergies in Your Nursling," vegetarianbaby.com.

126 Roberts, *Your Vegetarian Pregnancy,* 172

127 Ibid., 230.

128 Campbell and Campbell II, xv–368.

129 Wangen, "Food Allergy Solutions Review," FoodAlllergySolutions.com.

130 "Two New Studies Sour Milk's Image," pcrm.org.

131 Campbell and Campbell II, 6.

132 Ibid., 49–50.

133 Ibid., 6.

134 Barnard, "Nutrition and Prostate Health," cancerproject.org.

135 Robbins, *The Food Revolution,* 48.

136 Campbell, 178.

137 Robbins, *Diet for a New America,* 150.

138 Campbell and Campbell II, 292.

139 "What's Wrong with Dairy Products?" pcrm.org.

140 Kradjian, vegsource.com.

141 Epstein, *What's in Your Milk?* xxvi-xxvii.

142 Ibid., xxiii.

143 Ibid.

144 Ibid.

145 Ibid., 34.

146 Ibid.

147 Donohoe, "Letter to the Editor of Wall Street Journal—Long Standing Evidence of rBGH Dangers," organicconsumers.org.

148 Ibid., 7.

149 Kradjian, vegsource.com.

150 Gelles, *The Philadelphia Inquirer.*

151 Epstein, 34–35.

152 Donohoe, organicconsumers.org.

153 Green, "Not Milk: The USDA, Monsanto, and the U.S. Dairy Industry," LiPMagazine.

154 Kradjian, vegsource.com.

155 Cousens, 478.

156 Rauch, "Animal products in pregnancy," findarticles.com.

[157] Schuler, "Smart Meat and Dairy Guide for Parents and Children," iatp.org.

[158] Ibid.

[159] Ibid.

[160] Washam, "Suspect Inheritance. Potential Neurotoxicants Passed to Fetuses," ehponline.org.

[161] Greger, "Paratuberculosis and Crohn's Disease: Got Milk?" veganoutreach.org.

[162] Ibid.

[163] Ibid.

[164] Ibid.

[165] Ibid.

[166] Ibid.

[167] Ibid.

[168] Ibid.

[169] Kradjian, vegsource.com.

[170] Ibid.

[171] Ibid.

[172] Robbins, 150.

[173] Steinman, 122.

[174] Kradjian, vegsource.com.

[175] Cousens, 479.

[176] Campbell and Campbell II, xv–368.

[177] Epstein, 34-35.

[178] "What's Wrong with Dairy Products?" pcrm.org.

[179] Roberts, 173.

[180] Riley, 33 and McDougall, *The McDougal Program For Women*, 50.

[181] Robbins, 164.

[182] Holford, 42.

[183] Robbins, *The Food Revolution*, 101.

[184] Ibid., 107.

[185] Ibid.

[186] "Men and Osteoporosis," nof.org.

[187] "Calcium and Strong Bones," pcrm.org.

[188] Ibid.

[189] Ibid.

[190] Weiss, 87.

[191] "Egg Consumption Linked to Risk of Type 2 Diabetes," pcrm.org.

[192] "Incident Heart Failure Is Associated with Lower Whole-Grain Intake and Greater High-Fat Dairy and Egg Intake in the Atherosclerosis Risk in Communities (ARIC) Study," *Journal of the American Dietetic Association.*

[193] Saxe, "Ask the Doctor," cancerproject.org.

Endnotes

[194] Ibid.

[195] Ibid.

[196] Eisnitz, *Slaughterhouse,* 20.

[197] Ibid, 66.

[198] Ibid., 69-70.

[199] Ibid., 126-133.

[200] Ibid., 29.

[201] Ibid., 20, 28-29.

[202] Ibid., 71.

[203] Ibid., 166.

[204] Ibid.

[205] Ibid.

[206] Ibid.

[207] Ibid., front jacket.

[208] Ibid., 124.

[209] Ibid., 82.

[210] Ibid., 125.

[211] Ibid., 87.

[212] Ibid., 84.

[213] Ibid., 91.

[214] Ibid., 93.

[215] Ibid., 130.

[216] Ibid., 132.

[217] Ibid., 132-133.

[218] Ibid., 144-145.

[219] Ibid., 145.

[220] Ibid., 93.

[221] Ibid., 133.

[222] Ibid., 140-141.

[223] Ibid., 172.

[224] Ibid.

[225] Ibid., 173.

[226] Ibid., 174.

[227] Ibid., 175.

[228] Leake, "The rich emotional & intellectual lives of cows."

[229] "The Hidden Lives of Chickens," Peta.org.

[230] Rossella Lorenzi, "Study: Chickens Think About Future," animal.discovery.com.

[231] "Pigs: Smart Animals at the Mercy of the Pork Industry," Peta.org.

[232] "Fish Feel Pain," Fishinghurts.com.

[233] "Free-Range Eggs and Meat: Conning Consumers?" Peta.org.

[234] "Investigation Reveals Slaughter Horrors at Agriprocessors," Peta.org.

[235] Eisnitz, "Ask the Experts," Peta.org.

[236] Eisnitz, *Slaughterhouse,* 125.

[237] Chuck Jolley, "Hallmark/Westland Might Not Be An Anomaly

According To An OIG Report," CattleNetwork.com.

238 Brown, e-mail.

239 "Animal Friendly Quotes," Peta.org.

240 "Vegetarian 101," GoVeg.com.

241 "Factory Farming: Environmental Consequences," Animalalliance.ca.

242 Friedrich, e-mail.

243 "Livestock a major threat to the environment," fao.org.

244 Friedrich, e-mail.

245 Bruce Friedrich, "Taking the Food Crisis Personally," huffingtonpost.com.

246 Cook, "Environmental Hogwash," inthesetimes.com.

247 Friedrich, "Taking the Food Crisis Personally."

248 Ibid.

249 Ibid.

250 Ibid.

251 Cousens, 442.

252 Young, 82-3.

253 Howell, *Enzyme Nutrition,* 4.

254 Ibid., 4-5.

255 Cousens, 299.

256 Cichoke, *Enzymes & Enzyme*

257 Roberts, 69.

258 "Protein: Moving Closer to Center Stage," hsph.Harvard.edu.

259 Cichoke, *Enzymes & Enzyme Therapy,* 314.

260 Ibid., 417.

261 Holford, *The Optimum Nutrition Bible,* 29.

262 "How can I get Enough Protein? The Protein Myth." pcrm.org.

263 Ibid.

264 Cousens, 312.

265 Ibid.

266 Holford, 41.

267 Cousens, 587.

268 "Race Results Powered by Raw Food," runningraw.com.

269 "Vegan Athlete—Summary of vegan/vegetarian," veganathlete.com.

270 Michael Parrish, "Famous Olympic Wrestler Sushil Kumar Promotes Vegetarian Lifestyle With PETA," ecorazzi.com.

271 "Vegetarian and Vegan Famous Athletes," Veggie.org.

272 "Famous Vegetarians," happycpw.net.

Therapy, 105.

Endnotes

[273] "Vegan Ultimate Fighter Ricardo Moreira," mmacoverage.com.

[274] "World Vegan Day is November 1," healthline.com.

[275] Joshua Katcher, "Lean & Green: Jake Shields," thediscerningbrute.com.

[276] Jeff Caplan, "Go-To and Tofu Guy: Stack Makes Switch," star-telegram.com.

[277] Jonah Keri, "Who says you have to eat meat to be a successful athlete?" sports.espn.go.com.

[278] "Heather Moore, "Vegetarian Athletes At the Top of Their Games," gather.com.

[279] Thomas J. Billy, "FSIS Case Study—Meat and Poultry HACCP," fsis.usda.gov, and email from Jack Norris to Bruce Friedrich, November 27, 2002.

[280] "3/4 Chickens Bought Nationwide Harbor Salmonella or Campylobacter," organicconsumers.org.

[281] "Eggs Non Gratis," The Civil Abolitionist, weblinknn.com.

[282] "Top 10 Reasons Not To Eat Chickens,"goveg.com.

[283] "E. Coli Infection." American Academy of Family Physicians, Familydoctor.org.

[284] "3/4 Chickens Bought Nationwide Harbor Salmonella or Campylobacter," organicconsumers.org.

[285] Friedrich, e-mail.

[286] Freedman and Barnouin, *Skinny Bitch,* 44-45.

[287] Gelles, "Why Antibiotics in Meat Should Give You Pause," *The Philadelphia Inquirer*.

[288] "Drug-Resistant Bacteria Found in U.S. Meat," Reuters Medical News, 24 May 2001.

[289] Williams, "'What's in the Beef?' Interview with Howard Lyman, author of *Mad Cowboy*. Discussion of health aspects of additives in beef," Encyclopedia.com. and Williams, R.M., TLfDP #203, 26–27 (endnote).

[290] Friedrich, e-mail.

[291] "Union of Concerned Scientists Food & Farming Newsletter," organicconsumers.org.

[292] Friedrich, email.

[293] Roberts, 169.

[294] Williams, "What's in the Beef?" and Epstein, *The Politics of Cancer,* encyclopedia.com.

[295] Williams, "What's in the Beef?" and Sherman, *Life's Delicate Balance,* encyclopedia.com.

[296] Williams, "What's in the Beef?" and Epstein, *The Politics of Cancer,* encyclopedia.com.

[297] Williams, "What's in the Beef?" and Epstein, *The Politics of Cancer,* encyclopedia.com.

[298] Holford, 40.

[299] Schlosser, "The Cow Jumped Over the U.S.D.A," *New York Times*, commondreams.org.

[300] Ibid.

[301] Coupe, "Editorial: Mad Cows, Lunatic Politicians, & The Case for Traceback," cattlenetwork.com.

[302] "USTR demands Japan lift beef import restrictions linked to cow age," Japan Today, japantoday.com.

[303] Barnard, "Meat Too Tough to Eat," Hartford Courant, pcrm.org.

[304] "Environmental Facts," kingwoodgreeninfo.org.

[305] Williams, Rose Marie, "'What's in the Beef?'(Interview with Howard Lyman, author of *Mad Cowboy*. Discussion of health aspects of additives in beef),"

Encyclopedia.com.

[306] Roberts, 148 and 207.

[307] "A Cesspool of Pollutants. Now Is the Time to Clean-Up Your Body," nealhendrickson.com.

[308] "Silent Spring II," www.thirdworldtraveler.com.

[309] "Silent Spring II," www.thirdworldtraveler.com.

[310] "A Cesspool of Pollutants. Now Is the Time to Clean-Up Your Body," nealhendrickson.com.

[311] "Salmon farms producing tainted fish-farmed salmon not as healthy as wild salmon and fish farming industry pollutes the ocean," *New York Times*, findarticles.com.

[312] Ferdowsian, and Levin, "Fish Still Not a Healthy Choice," *The Providence Journal*, pcrm.org.

[313] Hooper, "Risks and benefits of omega 3 fats for mortality, cardiovascular disease and cancer: systemic review," *British Medical Journal*, bmj.com.

[314] Ferdowsian and Levin.

[315] Ibid.

[316] Riley and Nelson, 90.

[317] Roberts, 67-68.

Endnotes

318 Weil, Natural Health, *Natural Medicine,* 30.

319 Robbins, "What about Soy?" foodrevolution.org.

320 Jess Halliday, "Study links low sperm with high soy consumption," foodnavigator.com.

321 Mills, "Health benefits of soy-why the controversy?" womentowomen.com.

322 Roberts, 35.

323 Mills, womentowomen.com.

324 Roberts, 35.

325 Robbins, "What about Soy?" foodrevolution.org.

326 Mills, womentowomen.com.

327 Robbins, "What about Soy?" foodrevolution.org.

328 Mills, womentowomen.com.

329 Osborne, Sally Eauclaire, "Does Soy Have a Dark Side?" *Natural Health,* findarticles.com.

335 Weil, "Does Soy Have a Dark Side?" drandrewweilselfhealing.com.

336 Young, 68.

337 Whitney and Rolfes, *Understanding Nutrition,* 8th ed., 130-31.

338 James Scala, *25 Natural Ways to Lower Blood Pressure,* 7.

339 Ibid.

340 "High Blood Pressure, (Hypertension)," pcrm.org.

341 Ibid.

342 Scala, 6.

343 Ibid., 7.

344 Ibid.

345 "High Blood Pressure, (Hypertension)," pcrm.org.

346 "High Blood Pressure," americanheart.org.

347 Campbell and Campbell II, 15.

348 Barbara Abel, "Men and Heart Disease: Take Lifestyle Cues from Women," healthlink.mcw.edu.

349 Campbell and Campbell II, 3.

350 "Cholesterol and Heart Disease," pcrm.org.

351 Ibid.

352 Esselstyn, 30.

353 Ibid.

354 Ibid.

355 "Cholesterol and Heart Disease," pcrm.org.

356 Ibid.

[357] Ibid.

[358] Ornish, *Eat More, Weigh Less,* xi, and Butler RN, Lewis MI, Hoffman E, Whitehead ED, "Love and sex after 60," *Geriatrics.* 1994;49(10):27-32.

[359] Campbell and Campbell II, 14.

[360] Ibid.

[361] Ibid., 147.

[362] Ibid., 152.

[363] Ibid., 152.

[364] Ibid. and JW Anderson, "Dietary fiber in nutrition management of diabetes," *Dietary Fiber: Basic and Clinical Aspects,* 343-360.

[365] Campbell, 177.

[366] Campbell and Campbell II, 178.

[367] Robbins, *The Food Revolution,* 48, and "Dairy Products Linked to Prostate Cancer." Health Professional follow up study April 5, 2000.

[368] Neal Barnard, M.D., "Milk and Prostate Cancer: The Evidence Mounts," pcrm.org.

[369] John McDougall, M.D., "Saving Yourself from Prostate (or Breast) Cancer," vegsource.com.

[370] Campbell, 178, and Giovannucci E. "Dietary influences of 1,25 (OH)2 vitamin D in relation to prostate cancer." *Cancer Causes and Control 9* (1998): 567-582.

[371] Campbell and Campbell II, 179.

[372] Barnard, "Prostate Cancer: Prevention and Survival," cancerproject.org.

[373] Ibid.

[374] Ibid.

[375] Chan, Stampfer, Ma, Gann, Gaziano, and Giovannucci, "Dairy products, calcium, and prostate cancer risk in the Physicians' Health Study," ajcn.org, and Campbell and Campbell II, 180-181.

[376] McDougall, "Saving Yourself from Prostate (or Breast) Cancer," vegsource.com.

[377] Steinman, 120.

[378] Ibid.

[379] Ibid.

[380] Robbins, 19, and Neal Barnard, M.D., *The Power of Your Plate,* 25-6.

[381] Campbell, 7.

[382] Esselstyn, 38-43.

[383] Raymond Francis, "Cancer —Turn It On, Turn It Off," revolutionhealth.com.

Endnotes

[384] Esselstyn, 38.

[385] Robbins, *The Food Revolution,* 48.

[386] Ibid, and Giovannucci E, "Tomatoes, Tomato-Based Products, Lycopene and Cancer," *Journal of the National Cancer Institute*, 91 (1999): 317-31.

[387] "Lycopene: Benefits, Side Effects, Sources and Supplements," health.learninginfo.org.

[388] Robbins, *The Food Revolution,* 48, and "Vegetables Lower Prostate Cancer Risk," *Journal of the National Cancer Institute* 92 (2000): 61-8.

[389] Barnard, "Prostate Cancer: Prevention and Survival," cancerproject.org.

[390] Ibid.

[391] "What Men Should Know About Low Testosterone," menshealthnetwork.org.

[392] Ibid.

[393] Jane Collingwood, "Emotions and Weight Affect Testosterone Levels," psychcentral.com.

[394] Chris Christian, "Increase Testosterone Levels," fitness.suite101.com.

[395] Ibid.

[396] "5 ways to boost your Testosterone Levels," healthandmen.com.

[397] Ibid.

[398] "Increase Testosterone Levels," fitness.suite101.com.

[399] Ibid.

[400] Ibid.

[401] Ibid.

[402] Lisa Jones, "Spray 'n' Wash," menshealth.com.

[403] "Male Fertility," acupuncture.rhizome.net.nz.

[404] Ibid.

[405] Ibid.

[406] Ibid.

[407] Ibid.

[408] Esselstyn, 309.

[409] Ibid.

[410] "Male Fertility," acupuncture.rhizome.net.nz.

[411] "Bad Breath, Foods and Eating," kissmegoodnight.com.

[412] Scala, 113.

[413] "Reduce Heart Disease Risk: Encourage and Prescribe Exercise for Your Patients," medscape.com.

[414] Dr. Joseph Mercola, "How Exercise Reduces Your Risk of

Prostate Cancer," mercola.com.

[415] "In Men, Exercise Benefits Prostate, Sexuality," medicalnewstoday.com.

[416] "Daily exercise dramatically lowers men's death rates," heart.org.

[417] "The Importance of Water for Athletes," fitsense.co.uk.

[418] Elizabeth Quinn, "Proper Hydration for Exercise—Water or Sports Drinks," about.com.

[419] Quinn, "Proper Hydration for Exercise—Water or Sports Drinks," about.com.

[420] Ibid.

[421] Ibid.

[422] Ibid.

[423] Ibid.

[424] Elizabeth Quinn, "Water Intoxication—Hyponatremia," sportsmedicine.about.com.

[425] Quinn, "Proper Hydration for Exercise—Water or Sports Drinks," about.com.

[426] D. Enette Larson-Meyer, PhD, RD, *Vegetarian Sports Nutrition,* 24.

[427] Lisa Dorfman, *Vegetarian Sports Nutrition Guide,* 16-17.

[428] Larson-Meyer, 25.

[429] Dorfman, 42.

[430] Ibid., 43.

[431] Brenda Davis and Vesanto Melina, *Becoming Vegan,* 246.

[432] Ibid., 249.

[433] Ibid.

[434] Ibid.

[435] Brendan Brazier, "The High Performance Vegan Athlete: It is Possible!", vegkitchen.com.

[436] Ibid.

[437] Davis and Melina, 248.

[438] Ibid.

[439] Larson-Meyer, 57.

[440] Davis and Melina, 248.

[441] Larson-Meyer, 61.

[442] Davis and Melina, 251.

[443] Ibid.

[444] Dorfman, 20.

[445] Davis and Melina, 252.

[446] Brazier, "The High Performance Vegan Athlete: It is Possbile!", vegkitchen.com.

[447] Davis and Melina, 253.

[448] Ibid.

[449] Dorfman, 146.

[450] Davis and Melina, 252.

Endnotes

[451] Kamen, *New Facts About Fiber,* 43-85.

[452] Ibid., 14.

[453] Ibid., 10.

[454] Holford, 109.

[455] "About USDA," U.S. Department of Agriculture.

[457] Schlosser, "The Cow Jumped Over the U.S.D.A," *New York Times,* commondreams.org.

[458] Simon, "The Politics of Meat and Dairy," earthsave.org.

[459] Langeland, "Tainted Meat, Tainted Money: Consumer groups decry coziness between government, agribusiness," *Colorado Springs Independent* online.

[460] Schlosser, "The Cow Jumped Over the U.S.D.A."

[461] Ibid.

[462] Ibid.

[463] "National Animal Identification System: Goal and Vision," U.S. Department of Agriculture APIS Veterinary Services.

[464] Ibid.

[465] "USDA Cover-Up of Mad Cow Cases," Food, Consumer and Environment News Tidbits with an Edge.

[466] "USDA won't stop use of illegal hormones in the veal industry: cancer rates skyrocket in humans," newstarget.com.

[467] Nestle, *Food Politics: How the Food Industry Influences Nutrition and Health,* 73.

[468] Ibid.

[469] "Common Dairy Digestive Under-Recognized and Under-Diagnosed in Minorities," Johnson & Johnson.

[470] Severson, Kim, "Dairy Council to End Ad Campaign That Linked Drinking Milk With Weight Loss," NYTimes.com.

[471] "Surgeon General Asks: Got Bones?" gotmilk.com.

[472] Simon, "Dairy Industry Propaganda: Tale of Two Mega-Campaigns," originally published on vegan.com.

[473] "Surgeon General Asks: Got Bones?"

[474] Severson, "Dairy Council to End Ad Campaign That Linked Drinking Milk With Weight Loss."

[475] "About USDA."

[476] "National School Lunch Program

Background,"
healthyschoollunches.org.

[477] Ibid.

[478] Ibid.

[479] "The National School Lunch
Program Background, Trends,
and Issues," ers.usda.gov.

[480] "Effects of Food Assistance and
Nutrition Programs on Nutrition
and Health: Volume 4, Executive
Summary of the Literature
Review," ers.usda.gov.

[481] Schlosser, *Fast Food Nation,*
219-20.

[482] Simon, "Misery on the Menu."

[483] Victor Oliviera, "The Food
Assistance Landscape: FY 2006
Annual Report," ers.usda.gov.

[484] Ness, "Organic Food: Outcry Over
Rule Changes that Allow More
Pesticides, Hormones," The San
Francisco Chronicle,
commondreams.org.

[485] "Organic Industry and Consumers
Celebrate USDA Reversal on
Non-Food National Organic
Standards," The Weston A.
Price Foundation,
westonaprice.org.

[486] Harris, "Organic Consumers
Association (OCA), the Nation's

Largest Organic Consumer
Group Denounces Degradation
of Organic Food Standards by
Congress," about.com.

[487] "Organic Industry and Consumers
Celebrate USDA Reversal on
Non-Food National Organic
Standards."

[488] Krebs, "USDA Accused of
Allowing 'Sham' Certifiers to
Participate in National organic
Program," The Agribusiness
Examiner.

[489] "OCA and Environmental Groups
Sue USDA to Enforce Strict
Standards: Environmental
Groups Back Harvey Lawsuit,"
Organic Business News,
organicconsumers.org.

[490] "Nation's Largest Organic Dairy
Brand, Horizon, Accused of
Violating Organic Standards,"
The Cornucopia Institute.

[491] Brownell, Kelly D., *Food Fight: The
Inside Story of the Food Industry,*
America's Obesity Crisis &
What We Can Do About It, 260.

[492] Green, "Not Milk: The USDA,
Monsanto, and the U.S. Dairy
Industry," *LiP Magazine.*

[493] Ibid.

[494] "The U.S. Food and Drug

Endnotes

Administration (FDA) and the glutamate industry," truthinlabeling.org.

495 "Food Additives," new-fitness.com.

496 "Banned as Human Food, StarLink Corn Found in Food Aid," Environmental News Service.

497 Greger, "Rocket Fuel in Milk," Dr.Greger.org.

498 Ibid.

499 Cook.

500 Ibid.

501 Schlosser, *Fast Food Nation,* 210-214.

502 Cook.

503 Barnard, *Breaking the Food Seduction,* 17-19.

504 Ibid.

505 Ibid.

506 Ibid., 20-21.

507 Ibid.

508 Ibid., 50-51.

509 Ibid.

510 Ibid.

511 Ibid., 52.

512 Ibid.

513 Ibid.

514 Ibid., 53.

515 Diamond, *Fit For Life II,* 245.

516 Barnard, 102.

517 Ibid.

518 Ibid.

519 Ibid.

520 Ibid.

521 Cousens, 231-32.

522 Ibid.

523 Van Straten, *Super Detox,* 12.

524 Cousens, 231-34.

525 Ibid., 232.

526 Van Staten, 13.

527 Cousens, 233.

528 Ibid., 234.

529 Ibid.

530 Ibid., 231.

531 Mindell, *Earl Mindell's New Vitamin Bible,* 39-127.

532 Campbell, 232.

533 Ibid.

534 Ibid.

535 Interview with Dina Aronson, MS, RD.

536 Ibid.

537 Ibid.

538 Ibid.

539 Ibid.

540 "Omega-3 fatty acids," umm.edu.

541 Esselsytn, 279.

542 Vincent, Beth, MHS, "The importance of DHA during pregnancy and breastfeeding," pregnancyandbaby.com.

543 Ibid.

544 Interview with Dina Aronson, MS, RD.

545 Ibid.

546 Ibid.

547 Boschen, "Cycles of the Body," thejuiceguy.com.

548 Weil, *Natural Health, Natural Medicine,* 17-18.

549 Holford, 24.

550 Farlow, 41-2.

551 "Salts that Heal and Salts that Kill," curezone.com.

552 "National Cattlemen's Beef Association Pays for Sadistic Anti-Vegan 'Study,'" vegsource.com.

553 "New Study shows being fit lowers risk of stroke," menwell.com.au.

554 Ibid.

555 Myss, *Anatomy of the Spirit,* 53-55.

556 Ibid., 56.

557 Coates, *Old MacDonald's Factory Farm,* 13.